Praise for *The Complete Family Guide to Addiction*

"Wow, someone finally gets it! As an addict with 13 years in recovery, this book gives me so much insight into addiction, codependency, and what I put my family through. It also reminds me what people did that helped me, and what didn't help. Every family member or friend of an addict should read this book! It brought back a lot of pain for me, but is so accurate and enlightening. It will help you save your loved one without ruining yourself in the process."　　　　—Taffy L., San Rafael, California

"If you care about someone with an addiction, this is the book you need. Families and friends often spend months or years of frustration trying to figure out what addiction is and what they can do about it. This highly practical book cuts right to the chase—explaining the most current research and clinical experience in plain English—and tells you everything you need to know."
　　　　　　　　　　　　　　　—Joseph P. Scholl, LICSW,
　　　　　　　　　　　attending social worker, McLean Hospital

"This greatly needed book is packed with invaluable information for loved ones of people who struggle with addiction. Often lost and left by the wayside in addiction treatment, families are now taken by the hand and offered understandable explanations of complex concepts, presented in an unbiased way. The book's compendium of resources is remarkable."　　　　—An̶ ̶ ̶ ̶ ̶ ̶ ̶,̶ ̶MS, RDN,
　　　　　　　author of *Inside* ...

"Accessible and comprehensive, this book equips you with the latest understanding of the shattering challenges of addiction. Whether it is your grown child, spouse, or other loved one who is afflicted, this book reveals the best ways to offer support."
—Robert Miranda Jr., PhD, Department of Psychiatry and Human Behavior, Brown University

"Families who are knowledgeable about addiction and its treatment are in a better position to help the person they love. Without 'taking sides,' this easy-to-understand book describes a wide range of treatment approaches and provides useful suggestions and strategies for dealing with common issues. As an addiction treatment specialist, I found many useful ideas for educating my clients and their families."   —Oscar G. Bukstein, MD, MPH, Department of Psychiatry, Boston Children's Hospital and Harvard Medical School

"Employing sensible, reader-friendly language, the authors give us a comprehensive, evidence-based primer on addictions, the challenges they pose for individuals and families, and the many treatment modalities currently available."
—Gabor Maté, MD, author of *In the Realm of Hungry Ghosts: Close Encounters with Addiction*

THE COMPLETE FAMILY GUIDE
TO ADDICTION

Also Available

Integrated Group Therapy for Bipolar Disorder
and Substance Abuse
Roger D. Weiss and Hilary S. Connery

THE COMPLETE FAMILY GUIDE TO ADDICTION

EVERYTHING YOU NEED TO KNOW NOW
TO HELP YOUR LOVED ONE AND YOURSELF

THOMAS F. HARRISON
HILARY S. CONNERY, MD, PhD

THE GUILFORD PRESS
New York   London

The information in this volume is not intended as a substitute for consultation
with healthcare professionals. Each individual's health concerns should be
evaluated by a qualified professional.

Library of Congress Cataloging-in-Publication Data

Names: Harrison, Thomas F., author. | Connery, Hilary Smith, author.
Title: The complete family guide to addiction : everything you need to know now
    to help your loved one and yourself / Thomas F. Harrison, Hilary S. Connery.
Description: New York : The Guilford Press, [2019] | Includes bibliographical
    references and index.
Identifiers: LCCN 2018050165| ISBN 9781462538546 (paperback) |
    ISBN 9781462539642 (hardcover)
Subjects: LCSH: Substance abuse. | Substance abuse—Family relationships. |
    Substance abuse—Treatment. | BISAC: SELF-HELP / Substance Abuse &
    Addictions / Alcoholism. | PSYCHOLOGY / Psychopathology / Addiction. |
    MEDICAL / Mental Health. | SOCIAL SCIENCE / Social Work. | RELIGION /
    Counseling.
Classification: LCC RC563 .H37 2019 | DDC 362.29—dc23
LC record available at https://lccn.loc.gov/2018050165

Contents

· · · · · · · · **V. WHAT TO EXPECT IN RECOVERY** · · · · · · ·

Introduction

FAMILY AND FRIENDS—
THE FIRST RESPONDERS
TO THE ADDICTION CRISIS

Addiction is ravaging our society, killing thousands of innocent people and destroying the lives of many others, including the family and friends who so often bear the brunt of addicts' problems. In recent years, we've slowly begun battling back against the illness. But in at least one key respect, we're doing it all wrong.

There's no question that we've made progress. Addiction is increasingly accepted as a disease, or at least as a brain disorder that's a complicated product of biological and environmental factors, rather than simply a moral failing. Scientists have advanced their understanding of how it affects the brain. Promising new treatments are being developed. A lot is happening in offices, laboratories, and medical clinics.

But very little attention is being paid to the home, where family members struggle every day to persuade addicts to get help, support them in their recovery efforts, and pick up the pieces of their own lives. And it's in the home, among family members, where the battle against addiction will ultimately be lost or won.

Addiction is not like other illnesses. When people develop a disease such as cancer, they typically acknowledge that they're sick, go to a doctor, and follow a course of treatment. But the essence of addiction is that the addict is in denial about the problem. Addicts go to enormous lengths to hide the fact that they can't control their behavior, both from themselves and from others. They don't want to get treatment; they want to continue using, and they often loudly and aggressively resist others' efforts to assist them. And even if they get help, they're incredibly tempted to throw their treatment plan overboard and relapse.

As a result, in a vast number of cases, it's family members and friends who make the difference—who finally push addicts into seeking help and who support them in recovery. Doctors and social workers get (and deserve) a lot of credit, but it's family members who are the unsung heroes of the addiction crisis. Family and friends are the true first responders; they're the ones who are on the front lines of the battle, and who suffer the emotional wounds. And if we want to solve our society's addiction problem, we need to focus our efforts on helping loved ones—giving them the tools and support they need to heal both the addicts and themselves.

It's been said that by the time addicts admit to needing help, they're halfway to recovery. It's also been said that treatment is only a first step; the real struggle begins when addicts leave treatment and have to function in the real world. So, if addiction were an American football game, the first half would consist of understanding the problem and getting the addict to acknowledge the need for help. Treatment would be the third quarter, and supporting the addict in recovery would be the fourth.

And here's the problem: We have a very well-trained team playing the third quarter—doctors, scientists, social workers, counselors, and other specialized professionals. But the rest of the game depends primarily on the efforts of family members and friends—raw recruits who not only lack training and information but never wanted to be involved in the contest in the first place. Until we educate loved ones about how to successfully help addicts and themselves, we can continue to have a terrific third quarter, but we're still going to lose the game.

The addiction crisis will never be solved solely from a policy think tank or a lab or a rehab facility. It will be solved by empowering family members to help their loved ones, one unique situation at a time.

And that's where this book comes in.

WHY THIS BOOK IS DIFFERENT

This book is the culmination of many years of work—of lived experience, extensive research, clinical practice, and listening to hundreds of families' stories in support groups for addicts and loved ones. Its goal is to provide families and friends with a practical guide to the problem and to arm you with all the information you need to understand what addiction is, cope with the real-life problems it causes, find the most suitable treatment plan, and give recovery the best chance to succeed.

There are many other books on addiction. But apart from highly technical scientific treatises, they tend to fall into three groups:

Memoirs written by recovering addicts or their families. These can make for compelling and even inspiring reading. However, they seldom answer the burning practical questions that people affected by addiction have. (Many books that purport to "explain" addiction are really just a collection of brief memoirs or stories grouped under general topic headings.)

Self-help books for addicts. Self-help books have been popular for decades, and it's no wonder that some authors have tried to adapt the genre for addiction. The problem, though, is that addiction really isn't a self-help illness. If you took a poll of a thousand recovering addicts and asked them what finally turned their lives around, the number who answered "reading a self-help book" would almost certainly be zero. That's not to say that these books can't occasionally be helpful or inspiring, but the odds of overcoming an addiction by reading a self-help book are about equal to the odds of being cured of cancer by listening to a motivational speaker.

Professional disputes. Addiction is a large problem, and it touches many professional disciplines. Occasionally, experts in these disciplines write books arguing why their perspective on the issue is the best one. As a result, there are entire books arguing that addiction is a disease, and entire books arguing that it isn't. A psychotherapist will write a book "debunking" the Twelve-Step model, and a behavioral psychologist will write a book attacking the psychotherapy model. And so on. These turf wars may be very interesting to professionals in the field, but they are usually of little help to families looking for practical answers.

This book has no interest in taking sides or arguing that there is one "right" way to think about the problem in areas where experts disagree. Addiction is highly complex. The reasons that someone becomes an addict are unique to each individual, and the path to recovery is also unique to each individual. This book will not tell you what road to take; rather, it will give you a complete roadmap of the landscape, so that you'll be empowered to decide for yourself which is the best route for you and your loved ones.

THIS BOOK WILL HELP YOU IF ...

The purpose of this book is to explain addiction and to help families and friends to deal with it successfully, because no matter how much the science advances, for the foreseeable future it's families and friends who will hold the key to the solution.

However, it's not just families and friends who will benefit. People who are struggling with addiction can also use this book to understand their situation and the resources that are available to help them. And people who are wondering if they might have an addiction can use it to get a better sense of the nature and depth of their potential problem.

Furthermore, the book can be used by anyone who needs to better understand how to deal with or provide guidance to an addicted person. This includes doctors, nurses, social workers, therapists, corporate managers, human resources professionals, and clergy, among others.

More specifically, here's how the book will help:

- Part I explains the science behind addiction—what's happening in the brain and why.
- Part II looks at the emotional side of the problem and how families are affected. It discusses how families, friends, and others can help and can cope.
- Part III discusses many of the real-world legal and practical issues that addicts often face and ways to keep them out of trouble—a topic of great importance to families that addiction books typically never discuss.
- Part IV provides a detailed overview of treatment options, of which there are many.
- Part V describes the recovery process and the most effective strategies to keep it going for the long term.
- Finally, the Resources at the back of the book offer places to turn for additional in-depth information on the many issues discussed here.

At this point in an introduction, it's tempting to provide some scary statistics—how many people suffer from addiction, how common it is in the population, how much it costs society in medical expenses and lost productivity, and so on. You can easily find research showing that 10 percent or more of the population suffers from some sort of addiction at some point. But these figures have to be taken with a large grain of salt. Because there's no one clear test to determine if someone is an addict, because there's a stigma to addiction such that many people who suffer from it don't report it, and because the effects of addiction on loved ones, employers, and others are often subtle and hidden, there's really no good way to quantify the exact extent of the problem or its cost to society.

In the end, though, what matters to most people is not precisely how much addiction affects the general population, but how it affects their own lives and families.

Addiction thrives in an atmosphere of misunderstanding and stigma. Confusion, denial, and isolation are its oxygen, the things that enable it to keep going. This may partly explain its prevalence, because as a society we very seldom look it squarely in the face—which only makes it stronger.

The best weapon against addiction is clear, accurate, and unbiased information. This book is designed to provide that information, to answer your questions, and to bring the problem out of the shadows so that we can finally understand it—and defeat it.

•   •   •

A *note about terminology*: This book frequently uses the words "addict" and "addiction." Increasingly, a number of experts in the field have come to believe that these terms have negative connotations and that they might contribute to the stigma around the problem and to discrimination against people who suffer from it. These experts have begun trying to use other terminology, such as "person with a substance use disorder." The authors of this book certainly have no intention of contributing to the stigma—in fact, the entire book is a determined effort to dispel it. But the book uses the words "addict" and "addiction" because there are as yet no generally accepted alternatives and because the words are easily understood and are the ones most commonly used by people who have substance use issues—and their families. (A more detailed discussion of the language used to describe the problem can be found in Chapter 5.)

I

WHAT IS ADDICTION?

1

A Bewildering Illness

Addiction is no ordinary problem. For both addicts and their families, it's the world's most bewildering, maddening, and frightening illness.

Addiction is bewildering because it doesn't seem to make any sense for people to have no control over their actions. Why would people continue to drink or use drugs when doing so leads to horrendous consequences—when it so often costs them their job and their friends, alienates their loved ones, gets them into legal trouble, and ruins their health?

Why don't they just stop?

It's usually easy to understand a physical disease because it's similar to a broken part on a car. The pancreas is supposed to regulate blood sugar, for instance, but in a person with diabetes it's broken and it doesn't work properly. It can even be fairly easy to understand a mental illness such as schizophrenia because in that case it's a different part of the body—the brain—that isn't working properly, and the person is out of touch with reality.

But addiction is bewildering because nothing about the addict's body seems to be broken, and in general, addicts *are* in touch with reality. They're usually completely aware of the choices they're making. They may know that they love their family, and yet their family feels hurt by their actions. They may know that they're losing their job, running out of money, and left with fewer and fewer good options in life.

9

They may know that they're slowly (or not so slowly) killing themselves. And yet they keep going.

Addiction is also bewildering because addicts seem to have free will about every other aspect of their life. They can decide what to wear and what to eat for breakfast. Many are high-functioning, and during the day they can hold down very responsible jobs as lawyers, businesspeople, firefighters, teachers, and so on. Their lack of free will is limited to one very specific choice.

Addiction is bewildering not just to loved ones, but to addicts themselves. They often have no idea why they do what they do.

Addiction is maddening because the solution seems so simple: *Just stop.* Addicts often say, "I desperately wish I could stop," and they mean it. But they can't.

Addiction is also maddening for loved ones because they're used to being able to influence a family member's behavior. Typically, loved ones do everything they can think of to try to get the addict to quit, ranging from "a good long talk" to bargaining, pleading, shaming, yelling, wheedling, threatening, and punishing. Over time, they usually come to realize that none of these things works.

The inability to stop the ongoing train wreck often leaves family members feeling hopeless, powerless, and frustrated. Sometimes they blame themselves. They also often feel personally rejected. "If she loved me, she'd quit," they think. And the problem is frequently worsened by the tendency of addicts to blame those closest to them for their problems.

Addiction is frightening because it involves a loss of free will, which we think of as an essential component of our personalities—one of the things that makes us *us*. We typically don't identify with our pancreas, so we can more easily accept that our pancreas doesn't work properly. But take away our free will, our ability to make decisions and express who we are, and we feel that we're losing our very selves.

Addiction is also frightening because it threatens to take away not just addicts' health, as other diseases do, but everything else that they and their families value along the way. Addiction doesn't just want to kill people. It first wants to strip them of their money, their jobs, their friends, their families, their homes, their social respect, their autonomy, their sense of meaning and purpose, and their ability to enjoy anything at all in life.

And *then* kill them.

For now, there is no cure for addiction. At best, it can be managed as a lifelong chronic condition, similar to diabetes. But the fact that it *can* be managed, and often is, is still an enormous advance. Far more treatment options are available now than in the past, including rehabilitation programs, psychotherapy, prescription drugs, and support groups. On their own or with treatment, many addicts are able to put the problem behind them for good, and many others are able to enjoy long periods of recovery.

While we can't magically cure addiction, we can make it less bewildering. To understand how the problem affects addicts and their families, and how best to approach treating it, a good place to start is to understand what precisely addiction is and how it affects the brain.

• • • • • • • 2 • • • • • • •

What Makes Someone an Addict, as Opposed to a Heavy Drinker or a Recreational User?

When does someone cross the line from being a social drinker or regular drug user to being an addict? Many people think the answer to that question is simple, but it isn't.

For instance, a lot of people would say the difference is that "an addict can't stop." But that's not exactly correct. Addicts can often stop using, sometimes for days at a time, or weeks, or even months. Many high-functioning addicts can keep their substance use in check well enough to hold down very responsible jobs. Many addicts are perfectly fine the great majority of the time and only occasionally go on binges.

A common myth is that you can determine whether someone is an addict based on the amount of consumption, but that's not true either. For instance, one person might have 15 or more glasses of wine every week and be perfectly healthy, whereas an alcoholic could actually consume a smaller amount overall. Nor does the regularity of consumption matter—a healthy person might drink something every night, while an addict might go for much longer periods without using.

Addiction is also not defined by the *extent* of someone's consumption. A college student might drink enough at a keg party to end up in the hospital, for instance, whereas an addict might be able to limit his or her intake enough that no one at work notices.

Many people think that addiction is the same thing as substance abuse, but it's not. For example, a businesswoman might have a lot to drink after work and get pulled over for drunk driving, or a college student might get blackout drunk and sleep with someone he didn't mean to, or a teenager might let her friends pressure her into getting high before a test. All these people are abusing substances, in that they're using bad judgment regarding them and causing harm to themselves and potentially others.

But a person can use bad judgment about alcohol or drugs and not be an addict. In fact, a person can use bad judgment about substances repeatedly, over a very long time, and still not be an addict.

So . . . what *is* addiction?

Addiction is a chemical process in the brain. This process changes the way the brain reacts to drugs, and it impairs the person's decision-making abilities, at least when it comes to using substances. As a result, addicts lose the ability to make rational judgments with regard to this particular aspect of their behavior.

For this reason, the key to understanding addiction is not that the person can't stop, but that the person can't freely choose whether to stop. It's not that addicts use bad judgment with regard to substances; it's that they generally use *no* judgment. They experience their actions as stemming from compulsion rather than choice.

That's not to say that addicts have no free will at all when it comes to alcohol or drugs. They have free will to some extent, and they can often exercise control over their actions in situations where the consequences are particularly severe. But their free will is impaired, and they frequently make choices and decisions that they would never make if their brain were working normally.

This impairment of the brain commonly produces a number of other traits that can distinguish addicts from people who are simply heavy drinkers or drug users.

For instance, while addicts may be able to avoid using substances for considerable periods or in situations where it's necessary, they usually have enormous difficulty regulating or moderating their consumption once they do start using. High-functioning alcoholics might get up every day and breeze past the liquor cabinet on their way to work, for example, but if they have a drink or two to relax in the evening, it will likely be extremely difficult for them to stop there and go off and do something else.

Another common trait is that addicts tend to have a blind spot when it comes to their own behavior. Because their decision-making ability is impaired, and they're not freely and deliberately choosing to do things that are destructive, they have a lot of trouble acknowledging and taking responsibility for the things they do that are harmful. Addicts find it much harder than recreational users to recognize when substances are having a deleterious effect on their own lives and on their families' lives.

For most healthy people, being pulled over for drunk driving or having a girlfriend or boyfriend break up with you over your drug patterns is a "wake-up call" that's liable to prompt a change in lifestyle. Addicts, however, are much more likely to deny the problems that result from their own behavior or to blame them on others. Addicts tend to get frequent wake-up calls—the problem is that they almost always sleep through them.

Because addiction is complicated, it can be difficult for family and friends to tell whether someone is truly addicted, especially in the early stages. It's hard to believe that someone who can hold down a job, go without using when necessary, and seem normal most of the time can really have such a debilitating problem. And there's no simple test that will give you a yes-or-no answer.

In addition, addicts themselves often become experts at covering up their behavior and deflecting blame. The result is that it can take many months or years to recognize addiction for what it is.

That's another reason addiction is such a bewildering illness: Family members often ask themselves, "How on earth did I not recognize it sooner?"

So . . . how exactly does addiction affect the brain, and why does it happen to some people and not to others? These questions are discussed in the next chapters.

3

How Addiction Affects the Brain

In recent years, scientists have been able to develop a very good model for how the addiction process works in the brain. Understanding this process can be extremely helpful to addicts and their families because it can allow them to recognize what's going on and grasp why addicts behave in the confounding ways they do.

All human beings have a system in their brains to reward certain actions with pleasure. For instance, we feel happy when we eat a good meal, win a financial reward, spend time with friends, or have sex. This has an evolutionary function. People who eat well, succeed in competition, develop companionship, and so on are more likely to stay alive and to pass on their genes to the next generation. As a result, our brains have developed a system that rewards us for these actions with pleasurable feelings and teaches us to engage in them repeatedly.

The main chemical that makes us feel good is a neurotransmitter called *dopamine*. We experience pleasure when dopamine is released in the nucleus accumbens, a cluster of nerve cells under the cerebral cortex. Scientists sometimes refer to the nucleus accumbens as the brain's pleasure center.

What does addiction do? It "hijacks" this process and misdirects it in a destructive way.

Addictive substances such as alcohol and drugs cause a sudden release of dopamine in the nucleus accumbens. Studies with laboratory rats have shown that alcohol, opioids, and tobacco can cause a release that is as powerful as what typically occurs with food or sex. Cocaine can cause a far more potent release. And a drug such as crystal methamphetamine can cause a release of dopamine that is 10 times more intense than what is typically experienced during sexual intercourse.

The release of dopamine caused by alcohol and drugs is not just potentially more powerful than that associated with food, money, or sex—it's also easier and more reliable. Typically, it takes a lot of effort to prepare a delicious meal, do a good job at work, or have a romantic relationship. With alcohol and drugs, this effort is eliminated—you can get the reward without the work. Also, the life activities that commonly lead to pleasure come with some risk—a relationship might not turn out well, for instance, or a business deal might fall through. Drugs and alcohol are much more reliable.

Dopamine isn't just associated with pleasure. Along with another neurotransmitter, glutamate, it plays a role in learning, memory, and motivation. In evolutionary terms, this is because your brain doesn't just want you to experience pleasure when you engage in certain species-promoting activities. It wants you to learn to associate the pleasure with those activities and motivate you to engage in them more.

In people who are susceptible to addiction, the brain learns to crave the reliable pleasure that comes from alcohol or drugs and to seek frequent repetition.

HOW THE BRAIN REACTS

Since alcohol and drugs can provide the brain with unusually large dopamine quantities and can do so on a regular basis, the result is that the brain begins to change many neural circuits associated with mood, motivation, and stress.

Our brain naturally tries to regulate itself and to keep everything in balance. In particular, dopamine receptors are in constant flux in terms of how many there are, how sensitive they are, how concentrated they are in certain parts of the brain, and so on. A brain that is inundated with drugs will automatically alter the way it works in order to adapt.

The first way the brain reacts is that it starts reducing dopamine activity in an effort to regulate the system so it doesn't become overwhelmed. The result? People can continue using the same amount of the drug, but over time, the amount of pleasure they experience from the drug decreases. This is called "developing a tolerance." Once a tolerance is developed, the person needs to take more of the drug to achieve the same effect.

Of course, the more of the drug a person takes, the more the brain responds by making structural changes that reduce pleasurable drug responses (and increase drug-related stress responses). Eventually, the person takes very large quantities of the drug but experiences very little pleasure as a result.

Unfortunately, these structural changes also greatly limit the person's ability to experience pleasure from normal stimuli. As a result, the things that in the past used to give the person fun and enjoyment— family, friends, hobbies, sports—have less and less appeal. The person gradually loses interest in everything else in life.

The brain, however, has learned to associate pleasure with the drug. Because of this, and because the person is getting no other enjoyment out of life, he or she begins to experience intense cravings for the drug. The actual drug is less and less capable of relieving the cravings, but the cravings get all the stronger as a result. Eventually the person is able to experience very little in life other than a need to relieve the cravings, even though doing so doesn't produce much at all in the way of pleasure.

MORE CHANGES IN THE BRAIN

At the same time that this is happening, changes occur in two other parts of the brain.

One part is the amygdala, which (among other things) works a bit like a radar scanner—it constantly looks at the environment, filtering out unimportant information and focusing on people, places, and things that are likely to lead to a goal. As the brain becomes hijacked, the amygdala becomes more and more focused on environmental cues that are associated with substance use. Gradually, the person's attention becomes almost exclusively preoccupied with getting and using substances.

The other part of the brain is the prefrontal cortex, which is sometimes said to regulate "executive" functioning. It makes decisions about what to do by weighing the evidence and considering the consequences, and it limits impulses from other parts of the brain. For example, you might get angry at someone and be tempted to hit the person. But your prefrontal cortex would consider the likely consequences of a fight, weigh the costs and benefits, and probably cause you to walk away instead. The prefrontal cortex is sometimes called the brain's impulse-control or "braking" system.

When a hijacked brain is craving a substance, this chemically changes the prefrontal cortex by causing it to give far more importance to drug-seeking behavior than it otherwise would. As a result, the person's free will and ability to make normal, rational decisions are impaired and overwhelmed. For instance, rather than making a rational choice as to whether substance use is more important than keeping a job, taking care of a child, or staying out of debt, an addict's prefrontal cortex will cause him or her to believe that obtaining a drug is the more necessary thing to do.

This, by the way, is why it's impossible to reason with addicts or argue them out of their behavior. Much of the time, addicts truly believe that they are acting based on the part of their brain that weighs the issues and makes the most appropriate choices. And they *are*—it's just that that part of the brain isn't working properly.

There's a medical term, *anosognosia*, that describes an illness that makes it difficult for people to realize that they have the illness. Common examples include schizophrenia and Alzheimer's disease. The term could be applied to addiction, although addicts often have some limited or variable awareness of their problem—their awareness is just heavily impaired.

Importantly, the prefrontal cortex continues developing through early adulthood, and it isn't completely matured in most people until about age 25. That's why teenagers often seem to have difficulty with impulse control and making wise long-term decisions—the part of their brain that regulates these things hasn't fully developed yet.

Unfortunately, this means that when someone starts using drugs as a teenager, it can be easier for the addiction process to occur because the prefrontal cortex isn't fully prepared to "brake" the dopamine-seeking behavior. A number of studies have shown that people who use substances at an early age are more likely to become addicted to them. In fact, people who use alcohol or other mind-altering drugs before the age of 16 can permanently alter their brain structure and neurocircuitry in a way that will make them more vulnerable to addiction throughout their lives.

IT GETS WORSE

Addiction is often considered to be a progressive condition. That means that, over time, unless it's treated, it tends to become worse and worse. That's not always the case—some people seem to be able to exist in a "holding pattern" for many years, and this is especially true for people who use alcohol or marijuana as opposed to other drugs. But all addicts face the risk that, unless they get treatment or find some other way to turn things around, the problem will eventually reach the sort of end-stage described earlier, where the person has no pleasure in life and little motivation to do anything but relieve the cravings.

At that point, many addicts experience utter misery and hopelessness. They have become enslaved to the drug, have no real quality of life, and see no way out.

Addiction isn't fatal in itself, but a number of addicts eventually die from substance use (such as through an overdose or liver disease) or from other causes made possible by the generally poor health that typically results from addiction.

Some addicts commit suicide. We actually don't know how many because unless there's clear evidence such as a suicide note, coroners generally consider deaths that are caused by an overdose or by combining alcohol and pills to be accidents. But in fact, many people who die this way may well have been deliberately looking for a way out, or simply have stopped caring whether they stayed alive or not. That's how terrible the illness can eventually become if it's not treated.

The good news is that a large number of treatments are available and that most of the chemical changes in the brain caused by addiction are reversible. It takes time, but a brain that is no longer being "hijacked" and overly stimulated with artificial sources of dopamine will gradually return to normal functioning. Of course, a brain that is susceptible to addiction will likely always be susceptible, and certain changes in learning and memory that occur during addiction will continue to make people more vulnerable to relapse in the future. For this reason, people getting over an addiction are usually advised to engage in complete abstinence from addictive substances. But a person who does abstain can eventually expect to once again lead a full, happy life.

HOW DO WE KNOW ALL THIS?

You might be wondering how we know for sure that addiction is the result of a chemical process in the brain. It's an interesting story. Substance abuse has existed for thousands of years, but it's only very recently that researchers have started to understand how it's connected to brain functioning.

In the early 1800s, a few scientists began speculating that alcoholics might be driven not simply by bad moral choices but by a sense of unavoidable compulsion—which might be akin to an illness. However, they had no real idea of what might be responsible for this process.

In the late nineteenth century, when the United States experienced widespread problems with the new drug morphine, scientists were confronted with a strange phenomenon: large numbers of lifelong upstanding citizens who were prescribed medicine for an ailment and soon underwent a personality change that made them extremely dependent on the drug. Furthermore, these "addicted" people tended to develop a number of highly specific common behavioral characteristics. This suggested the possibility that it wasn't just people who were abusing drugs—*the drugs might in some way be abusing people*, or at least be responsible for altering their behavior in ways they couldn't control.

In other words, scientists began to suspect that the problem wasn't people choosing to behave badly; it was the drugs themselves behaving badly in the ways they affected people.

In the twentieth century, scientists began testing this theory with mice, rats, and other laboratory animals. Sure enough, it turned out that researchers were able to get otherwise healthy animals addicted to drugs. Since laboratory mice don't have the same complicated free will that humans do, it appeared that the drugs themselves really were "addictive" and had a negative physiological effect.

Clearly, the mechanism by which addictive substances affected people's behavior must have something to do with the brain. But what? Science's understanding of how the brain works was still in its infancy. All that changed starting in the 1990s, when brain scans—including PET and MRI scans—began to be widely available for research.

As many scientists suspected, these scans showed that the brains of addicted people were significantly different from those of people who didn't have an addiction. The scans also let scientists see exactly *where* the differences were—generally in the circuits that involve pleasure, learning, memory, decision making, and motivation.

Through careful research, scientists were able to establish the precise mechanism by which drugs alter the brains of addicted people, overriding their normal thought processes and resulting in the unfortunate symptoms of addiction. They were also able to establish that the brains of people who stop abusing drugs are, for the most part, able to return to normal.

4

Why Do Some People Become Addicts and Others Don't?

Take two random people on the street. One of them can drink cock-tails, smoke marijuana, go to a casino, and take high-powered pain-killers and be perfectly fine. For the other, these actions lead to a down-ward spiral and a lifetime of misery. Why one and not the other?

This is a key unanswered question in addiction research. As you saw in the last chapter, scientists have a very good handle on how the addiction process happens in the brain. What they don't know is why it happens to some people and not to others.

Because there's no clear answer, lots of experts from lots of differ-ent fields have provided lots of different explanations. People who are experts in one particular field tend to see the solution through the prism of their own expertise. Often these explanations are in conflict.

For instance, neuroscientists tend to focus on the chemical changes in the brain. Many of them believe that *anyone* can become an addict if the person simply consumes enough substances to alter the brain's dopamine system.

Geneticists are more likely to believe that there's a genetic basis for the problem and that certain genes create susceptibility in certain people and not in others.

Many psychotherapists believe that substance abuse is triggered by life events, in particular by unresolved conflicts or trauma earlier in life.

But other therapists put less emphasis on past experiences and focus instead on a person's erroneous perceptions or ways of thinking in the present.

Politicians who write laws for a living often believe that addiction is a legal problem—that you can solve heroin addiction by making heroin illegal, for example. In effect, they say that addiction stems from a bad moral choice and should be a crime, like robbery or lying on your tax returns.

Many people believe that addiction is the result of a character flaw and that addicts are simply weak people who lack willpower.

And many Alcoholics Anonymous members will tell you that addiction is a spiritual problem and that an addict is someone who needs a changed relationship with a higher power.

With all these different voices offering different explanations and solutions, it's hard to know what to think.

The wisest answer may be that there is no one single explanation for why some people become addicts. Each person is unique, and each person comes to the problem in his or her own way. One person might turn to substance abuse because of a childhood trauma, while another might be seeking relief from problems in the present. One person might have a genetic susceptibility, while another is vulnerable because of having started drinking at age 12. There might be multiple causes within each person, and in some cases there might be no one clear predominant cause. But somehow, for each person who becomes an addict, the various risk factors come together in a "perfect storm" that results in addiction.

THE STRESS–VULNERABILITY MODEL

One way of talking about the "perfect storm" theory is what psychologists call the "stress–vulnerability model." This is a way of thinking about mental illnesses in general that first became popular in the 1970s. It wasn't specifically developed for addiction, but there are interesting parallels. The basic idea is that mental disorders result from a combination of biological susceptibilities and stress.

A good metaphor for this model is a water tank. Imagine that we all have a water tank inside us, with a pipe sending water in and another pipe taking water out. Our genes and other biological factors determine the size of the tank. The inflow pipe is stress—more water flows into the tank when we have a stressful environment. The outflow pipe represents our coping mechanisms. When we have good ways of dealing with stress and a lot of social support, we are able to take a lot of water out of the tank.

If there's a large tank, a limited amount of stress, and a well-functioning outflow pipe, people tend to be emotionally healthy. But if there's a small tank to begin with, a lot of stress, and a clogged outflow pipe, the tank may overflow, and the result is a mental illness.

A number of studies have confirmed that high levels of unrelieved stress tend to produce chemical changes in the brain that make mental illness more likely. For instance, stress hormones can cause stem cells that normally mature into neurons to turn into a completely different type of cell, which can affect the way that the parts of the brain that govern rational thinking communicate with the parts that govern learning and memory.

Interestingly, we tend to think of stress as a bad thing—it can result from losing a job, a relationship breakup, the death of a loved one, being a crime victim, and so forth. But it's important to remember that even positive experiences can be stressful. For instance, starting a new job or relationship or having a baby can be wonderful events, but they also tend to disrupt routines and cause anxiety.

Stress can also be the result of trauma or other issues in the past that we haven't fully resolved in the present.

Coping mechanisms can include exercising and getting enough sleep, a good diet, positive social skills, healthy leisure activities, and having trusted people to talk to about problems.

Applying this model to addiction would suggest that some people are born with a greater genetic or biological susceptibility to the addiction process in the brain and that, for them, addiction may be triggered by stressful situations or traumatic experiences along with limited coping abilities and environmental factors such as exposure to drugs.

Many purely physical diseases have a similar basis. For instance, it's widely believed that some people have a greater genetic susceptibility to cancer and that this vulnerability can be triggered by environmental factors such as smoking. People may also have a biological susceptibility to diabetes that can be triggered by behavior such as overeating.

THE ROLE OF GENES

Some research has strongly suggested that susceptibility to addiction has a genetic basis. For instance, studies have compared identical twins (who have the same genes) with fraternal twins. These studies show that if one twin becomes an addict, there's a much higher likelihood that an identical twin will become an addict than that a fraternal twin will.

Other studies of adopted children have shown that children are more likely to become addicts if one of their birth parents was an addict than if one of their adoptive parents was an addict.

This is persuasive evidence, but it doesn't identify which gene or genes cause the problem. In fact, no one has ever been able to identify an "addiction gene." Rather, the current thinking among geneticists is that there may be a multiplicity of genetic variants, all of which in one way or another make susceptibility to addiction more or less likely.

For instance, scientists have been able to isolate certain genetic combinations that are more or less common in alcoholics and cocaine addicts. They have also been able to show that mice bred with certain genetic combinations respond very differently to drug stimuli.

Another example is the fact that many Asian people have a genetic enzyme variant that causes unpleasant reactions when they drink alcohol, including headaches and nausea. Because of this, people with this genetic variant are much less likely to become alcoholics.

And it has been shown that the drug naltrexone, which is sometimes given to recovering alcoholics to reduce cravings, works more or less well depending on the person's genetic makeup.

However, genetics is not destiny. In fact, while the studies of identical twins show that one twin's becoming an addict makes it more likely that the other one will, it's still the case that if one twin becomes an addict, *most* of the time the other one won't—so even virtually identical genes won't produce the same result more than 50 percent of the time.

THE ROLE OF THE ENVIRONMENT

The fact that addiction can't be explained solely by genetics suggests that environmental factors play a very big part. One obvious environmental factor is simply the availability of the substance. For instance, people are less likely to become alcoholics if they grow up in a strict Mormon community where no one drinks alcohol and are less likely to become heroin addicts if they live in a remote area where heroin is hard to come by. On the other hand, a young person who has little parental supervision and lives somewhere where drugs are freely available at a nearby street corner is at much greater risk.

The fact that addiction correlates with availability can be seen generally from the fact that the two most widely abused substances in the English-speaking world—alcohol and tobacco—are also the most widely available, and from the fact that the opioid crisis in the United States followed directly on the heels of a dramatic increase in the number of opioid prescriptions. But there are also scientific studies that back this up. For instance, it's been shown that in two otherwise similar geographic areas, if one has a higher density of bars and liquor stores, it will also have a higher density of problem drinkers.

Consistent with the stress–vulnerability model, research has demonstrated that one of the principal environmental factors that affect addiction is stress. For instance, it has been shown that monkeys who are exposed to a stressful environment are much more likely to become addicted to cocaine.

There's a lot of research showing that traumatic experiences, particularly those that occur in childhood, correlate with mental health problems in adulthood—including addiction.

One of the most comprehensive such studies is the Adverse Childhood Experiences Study conducted in part by the U.S. Centers for Disease Control and Prevention. Researchers interviewed 17,000 people in the 1990s about childhood trauma and have followed them ever since to see how they fare through their lives.

The study defines an adverse childhood experience, or ACE, as mental, physical, or sexual abuse; emotional or physical neglect; witnessing domestic violence; having parents who get a divorce; or having a parent who is mentally ill, addicted, or in jail.

One follow-up survey found that every single type of ACE correlates with a higher risk of alcoholism in later life and that having multiple ACEs increases the risk by two to four times. Another survey found that people who reported five or more ACEs were 7 to 10 times more likely to develop an addiction.

Although the ACE study was conducted in the United States, these types of results are not limited to Americans. For instance, a study in

Sweden found that children had twice the risk of developing an addiction later in life if they lost their parents, witnessed domestic violence, or had a parent diagnosed with cancer.

Sometimes genetic factors and childhood trauma are hard to separate. For instance, one study found that people who had a parent who was an addict were eight times more likely to become addicts themselves. However, it's unclear what part of this was due to the child's genetic inheritance and what part was due to the fact that having an addicted parent is itself a traumatic experience.

Of course, everyone is different. Many people with "good" genes become addicted, and many people with "bad" genes don't. Likewise, many people escape childhood trauma unscathed, while numerous addicts report having had happy, trouble-free childhoods. There's no one combination of factors that produces the "perfect storm."

Not everyone agrees with the stress–vulnerability model, and while many studies seem to support parts of it, there's no hard scientific proof that it explains mental illness in general or that it applies to addiction in particular. Scientists who question the model often note that proving it would be extremely difficult, since there's no easy way to quantify scientifically how much stress people experience or how good their coping skills are.

Nevertheless, the model can be a helpful way of thinking about addiction. And it's clear that reducing stress in addicts' lives and supporting their coping mechanisms can only help in recovery.

IS THERE AN "ADDICTIVE PERSONALITY"?

Another question that arises frequently is whether some people simply have a personality that is prone to addiction.

Some professionals who work in the field say that in their experience there is a personality type that very frequently—not always, but very frequently—is found in people who suffer from addiction. A large number of addicts report that, growing up, they felt a great deal of anxiety. They tended to feel socially awkward, depressed, sensitive, worried, inadequate, out of place, and lacking in self-esteem and a sense of self-worth. While these feelings might be connected to a difficult childhood, they often seem to have arisen on their own.

Of course, *all* teenagers tend to feel moody and socially awkward. The difference is that these people tended to feel this way all the time and to continue feeling this way even in the face of social or academic successes that would have made other young people confident or proud.

This is sometimes called the "hole in the soul" theory—the idea that people who become addicts are missing something in their personality that makes other people feel confident, relaxed, and happy.

A large number of addicts report that when they first used a substance, it was as though the hole in their soul magically went away. They no longer felt anxious; they felt happy and confident. Often, they say, they felt good for the first time in their lives.

As a result, they wanted to use the substance again and again.

Not everyone accepts the idea that there's an addictive personality. It's obviously impossible to prove scientifically that someone has a hole in his or her soul, and even the concept of "personality" itself is hard to define apart from the combination of biology and environment. Behavioral psychologists in particular tend to argue that there's no scientific proof that people who become addicts have a consistent personality pattern prior to becoming addicted. They often suggest that what appear to be personality traits associated with addiction might in fact just be symptoms of the addiction itself.

That may be true, although it's also possible that genetic variants that produce a susceptibility to addiction are related to certain temperamental traits that are anecdotally associated with addicts. The relationship between genes and personality is hopelessly complicated and difficult to untangle.

Another thing to consider is that the hole in the soul might not be a personality trait at all; it might be an undiagnosed mental illness. People who have other types of mental illness are much more likely than the general population to develop an addiction. Common mental illnesses that coincide with addiction include depression, anxiety disorders, personality disorders, attention-deficit/hyperactivity disorder, and posttraumatic stress disorder. Any of these disorders could, in the right circumstances, be mistaken for a "hole in the soul."

When a person has both an addiction and a separate mental illness, these are called "co-occurring disorders." (Co-occurring disorders are discussed in more detail in Chapter 32.)

While the hole-in-the-soul idea can't be proven scientifically, it's surprising how often the concept resonates with family members of addicts. One reason might be that it helps to describe how substances seem to "work" differently for addicts than for other people.

For most people, drugs and alcohol make them feel "high"—they get a sense of relaxation, excitement, bliss, and creativity that's above and beyond their normal life. It's fun for a while, but they're also content to return to the real world so they can take care of life's necessities.

For addicts, though, while drugs and alcohol produce pleasure, they don't necessarily make them feel "high" in the same way they do for other people. However crazy it might seem, addicts commonly use drugs and alcohol because they make them feel *normal*.

Healthy people can enjoy the dopamine rush associated with a substance, but also see it as an unusual event that needs to be managed through reasoned decision making. They generally feel good; the substance just briefly makes them feel extra-good. Addicts, however, may typically feel bad, and the substance makes them feel as though they have finally achieved equilibrium and normality. This can make it much more likely that they will continue using it even in ways that would strike others as irrational.

So Is Addiction a Disease?
(and If Not, What Is It?)

There are a lot of ways of thinking about addiction. In recent years, many people have started calling it a disease.

The usual definition of a disease is a disorder of a structure or function in the body that isn't caused by a physical injury. Since addiction causes an unhealthy rewiring of the brain, it sure seems like a disease.

Nevertheless, to fully understand addiction, it's worth looking just a bit at how the problem has been regarded in the past and why some people *don't* consider it a disease.

ADDICTION AS A MORAL FAULT

In ancient times, addiction was sometimes thought of as a kind of demonic possession. This is in some ways a very powerful description. Anyone who has ever dealt with a family member in the throes of an active addiction will probably tell you that it appears as though the person he or she knows and loves has somehow been replaced by an evil demon.

But over time, many people came to view it as a moral fault or a character defect. After all, it certainly *appears* as though an addict is simply making bad moral choices—getting drunk instead of going to work, gambling away the family's money, or otherwise acting irresponsibly. In the nineteenth century, a common medical term for alcoholism was "intemperance"—implying that it was a vice, the opposite of the virtue of temperance.

A lot of people still feel this way. And even people who think of addiction as a disease still often subconsciously blame addicts for their behavior.

In many places, the moral fault theory led to a public policy approach in which the government banned substances used by addicts and criminalized their behavior. For instance, alcohol was illegal in the United States from 1920 to 1933, and even today most U.S. states ban public drunkenness and open containers of alcohol. The United States criminalized heroin in 1924 and marijuana in 1937. (Gambling, consuming pornography, and other arguably addictive behaviors have also long been regulated. These behaviors are discussed in Chapter 7.)

Today some U.S. states have legalized marijuana, but it is still illegal at the federal level, as are other substances such as cocaine, heroin, and methamphetamines.

Overall, it can be said that the public policy of the United States reflects complex health and safety concerns, including profiteering and the social costs and harms of substance abuse, but in general views addiction as a moral fault—the type of misconduct that can be punished as a crime, similar to burglary or assault.

Of course, some people who support antidrug laws don't consider addiction to be simply bad behavior. They believe that addiction is a disease, but they think that antidrug laws will help to stop the disease, by preventing people from starting to use a drug or from continuing to use it.

The objection to this theory is that the threat of arrest is of limited value as a deterrent when a person's free will is impaired by addiction and the person can't make deliberate, rational choices. If addicts aren't deterred by the possibility of losing their job, losing their home, losing their loved ones, or losing their own life, it's unlikely that the additional threat of arrest will solve the problem. And while a prison term might physically separate addicts from their substance of choice, it does nothing to address their underlying dependency.

ADDICTION AS A DISEASE

Starting in the 1940s, when Alcoholics Anonymous first became popular, the view of addiction started to change. Rather than treating alcoholics simply as bad people, AA viewed them as having a spiritual sickness. AA also spoke of alcoholism as a physical condition, perhaps similar to an allergy. Most important, AA offered a *treatment*—a process alcoholics could undergo to get better. And in many cases it worked.

The idea that alcoholism wasn't just bad behavior but an actual condition that could be treated gave rise to the disease model—the concept that addiction was something that people "came down with" and that they could be helped.

Doctors responded. The New York City Medical Society on Alcoholism was founded in 1954 and became the model for professional organizations devoted to addiction medicine. In 1956, the American Medical Association officially declared alcoholism to be a disease.

The disease model took off further in the 1990s when scientific research began to show that addicts underwent specific chemical changes in the brain as the addiction process progressed. Because addiction appeared to be the result of a part of the body (the brain) not working as it should, it seemed more and more like a traditional medical disease, such as diabetes or cancer.

And the disease model was reinforced even more when drugs began to come onto the market to treat alcoholism and opioid abuse. If it can be treated with drugs, people thought, it must be a medical disease.

ADDICTION AS A PSYCHOLOGICAL DISORDER

At the same time that a biological basis was being found for addiction, psychologists also began to treat it.

The "bible" of psychiatric diagnosis in the United States, which lists all the psychological disorders and their criteria, is the American Psychiatric Association's *Diagnostic and Statistical Manual of Mental Disorders*, now in its fifth edition (called *DSM-5*). *DSM-5* doesn't refer to "addiction" and doesn't call it a "disease." Instead, it describes something called "substance use disorder."

A big difference between traditional medicine and behavioral health care (psychology, psychiatry, social work, behavioral health nursing, etc.) is that traditional medicine usually defines diseases in terms of biological changes within the body, whereas psychology typically defines disorders based on outward behaviors and patients' reports of their thoughts and moods. So, for instance, *DSM-5* lists 11 characteristics, almost all of them outward behaviors or inner experiences, and says that you suffer from a substance use disorder if you have some or all of them. (It doesn't matter what's happening with your brain chemistry.)

Generally, the 11 criteria involve people using a substance more than they intended, using it in a way that takes up a great deal of their time, and using it even though it causes problems at work or in social relationships. A substance use disorder is considered mild, moderate, or severe depending on how many of the criteria the person meets.

Whenever someone is "diagnosed" with a substance use problem in the United States (for treatment or insurance purposes), the diagnosis is based on the 11 criteria in *DSM-5*. In most other countries, the diagnosis is based on the criteria in the World Health Organization's *International Classification of Diseases*, often called *ICD-10*. *ICD-10* criteria differ slightly but are very similar.

MODERN CRITICISM OF THE DISEASE MODEL

In recent years, a number of experts have criticized the disease model.

For instance, in the book *The Biology of Desire*, neuroscientist Marc Lewis claims that addiction is really just a habit. He says it's true that addiction rewires the brain, but lots of habits rewire the brain. Indeed, the brain is highly plastic and adaptable, and all sorts of behavioral and environmental factors change the way the brain functions all the time. For this reason, he says, addiction shouldn't be considered a disease, but rather a maladaptive behavior or a developmental problem.

Some psychologists have noted that addiction affects people in tremendously different ways. While lung cancer tends to be a known process with clear treatment protocols, for example, addiction is far more variable and far more susceptible to environmental cues. Therefore, they say, it can't just be reduced to a biological illness.

Some experts even argue that treating addiction as a disease makes it harder for addicts to get better.

When most people say "addiction is a disease," they intend to be compassionate. They are saying that it's a disease *as opposed to a moral fault*, and so the addict shouldn't be blamed for it. However, these experts argue that treating addiction as a disease rather than as a habit that can be overcome has the effect of increasing the stigma of addiction, making addicts feel helpless, and discouraging them from making needed changes in their lives.

Today, a number of experts don't even like to use the term "addiction" because they think it's loaded with negative connotations. They prefer to say "substance use disorder" or use some other language. Indeed, the authors of the book *Beyond Addiction* argue that it's better not to try to classify or explain the problem at all and to simply focus on changing behavior related to substances.

So what is addiction, really? Perhaps the best way to describe it is that it's *an impaired ability to make healthy choices regarding a substance or behavior, which is associated with chemical changes in the brain.*

For simplicity, this book often uses the words "addiction," "addict," and "disease" because they are common terms that are widely understood. But obviously, as with most things associated with addiction, the truth can be very complicated.

6

Why Do People Get Addicted to One Particular Substance and Not Others?

Why do some people become alcoholics, some become heroin addicts, some become addicted to cocaine, and so on?

Science doesn't have a good answer to this question. Whatever the underlying problem that causes addicts to turn to substances in the first place, they usually find that certain substances work better for them than others in alleviating it. But there's no conclusive research as to why this is.

Most addicts have what's called a "drug of choice." Alcoholics, for instance, tend to stick to alcohol and are unlikely to one day suddenly try substituting something else.

However, this is merely a general rule, and there are exceptions. Some people start with one drug of choice and migrate to another one if they find that it makes them feel better. Some people have multiple addictions—one person might be both a gambling addict and an alcoholic, while another is an alcoholic and a cocaine addict. Some people have a drug of choice but are willing to substitute a similar drug if their drug of choice becomes hard to find or too expensive. And a small number of people seem to have no particular preference and are happy to take whatever drug they can get their hands on.

One explanation for why addicts have a particular drug of choice has to do with availability and habit. For instance, alcohol and nicotine are by far the most abused drugs in the United States, and they're also the most readily available. They're legal, they can be obtained almost anywhere, and they're more or less ubiquitous in the culture.

Almost everyone drinks alcohol at some point, so if a person has an addictive tendency, alcohol has a good chance of bringing it out. Once people get hooked on alcohol, they may stick with it simply because they're used to it, they know it works, and it's easy to get.

In a similar way, people who have been prescribed a powerful painkiller due to cancer, surgery, or chronic pain may develop an addiction as a result of being exposed to the drug. It's no coincidence that the enormous increase in painkiller prescriptions over the last few decades has been accompanied by an enormous increase in painkiller addiction.

Another possible explanation is that while all addictive substances tend to have one thing in common, which is that they trigger a sudden release of dopamine in the brain, they have differing secondary effects and may make people feel different in other respects. In fact, drugs tend to fall into different "families" depending on how they otherwise affect the brain and how they make people feel. So the reason that addicts prefer one substance over another may lie in how they react to these secondary effects. An argument for this theory is that it might explain why someone would become addicted to cocaine, for instance, even though alcohol is far cheaper, is far easier to get, and doesn't carry heavy criminal penalties.

Another argument for this theory is that it explains why so many people who get addicted to prescription painkillers eventually migrate to heroin—which is part of the same drug family.

There are three main drug families when it comes to addiction—depressants, stimulants, and opioids. Hallucinogens are also widely abused, but they are less likely to result in addiction because their effect on the brain's dopamine processing is different. Alcohol and marijuana don't fit perfectly into any of these categories and are discussed separately later in the chapter.

DEPRESSANTS

Depressants are drugs that slow down the central nervous system and generally lessen brain activity. They can reduce a person's nervousness and inhibitions and are commonly prescribed to treat anxiety, panic disorders, insomnia, and sometimes seizures.

The most common (and dangerous) kind of depressants are benzodiazepines, often known as benzos. Many people develop addictions to benzos even while they are taking them at prescription-level doses. Users can develop a high tolerance for benzos very quickly. Withdrawal symptoms can be severe, and sudden withdrawal can in some cases cause seizures that may be fatal. (Because of the risk of seizures, benzos and alcohol are the two substances for which it is most important to detox in a medically controlled environment.)

Benzos commonly prescribed for anxiety disorders include diazepam (Valium), alprazolam (Xanax), lorazepam (Ativan), clonazepam (Klonopin), chlordiazepoxide (Librium), oxazepam (Serax), and clorazepate (Tranxene).

Benzos commonly prescribed for seizure disorders include diazepam (Valium), clonazepam (Klonopin), lorazepam (Ativan), and clorazepate (Tranxene).

Benzos commonly prescribed for insomnia include triazolam (Halcion), temazepam (Restoril), quazepam (Doral), and estazolam (ProSom).

Since many people who become addicts suffer from underlying feelings of anxiety and worry, it's easy to see why benzos could become their drug of choice.

Barbiturates are another type of depressant that can be abused. These drugs were widely prescribed in the 1960s and 1970s for anxiety and insomnia, but today they have largely been replaced by benzos. The most commonly abused barbiturates are amobarbital (Amytal), pentobarbital (Nembutal), secobarbital (Seconal), and Tuinal (a combination of amobarbital and secobarbital).

STIMULANTS

Stimulants increase activity in the central nervous system in adults, reducing fatigue and creating a sense of mental alertness, high energy, and exhilaration. In addition to triggering a dopamine surge, they increase production of norepinephrine, which can raise a person's heart rate and blood pressure and thus create an energy boost.

Cocaine is a stimulant, as are amphetamines, methamphetamines (such as crystal meth), and synthetic cathinones (better known as bath salts).

Curiously, some of the same drugs that create high energy in adults often have the opposite effect on children. In children, these drugs work to stimulate nerves that slow down other overactive nerves, producing a calming effect.

As a result, some of these drugs are prescribed for children who have been diagnosed with attention-deficit/hyperactivity disorder. Common drugs used for this purpose include methylphenidate (Ritalin and Concerta), dextroamphetamine (Dexedrine), pemoline (Cylert), and Adderall (a combination drug).

Stimulants can also be used as an appetite suppressant. Drugs used for this purpose include phendimetrazine (Bontril and Prelu-2), phentermine (Pro-Fast, Ionamin, and Adipex-P), benzphetamine (Didrex), and diethylpropion and amfepramone (Tenuate).

Many people start off taking these drugs for medically appropriate reasons but become addicted.

Stimulants might well become the drugs of choice for people whose jobs require staying alert for long periods or having peak alertness at specific periods.

Caffeine qualifies as a stimulant, by the way. So does nicotine, although research using EEG monitoring has shown that nicotine can also act as a depressant.

OPIOIDS

Opioids, also called narcotic analgesics, are powerful painkillers used to treat acute pain such as from cancer or surgery. They are typically prescribed for limited periods of fewer than 30 days. They can produce feelings of emotional well-being, a sense of detachment, and a dreamy euphoria.

Common opioid drugs include oxycodone (OxyContin, Percocet, Percodan, Roxiprin, and Roxicet), meperidine (also known as pethidine and sold as Demerol), hydrocodone (Vicodin, Norco, Lorcet, and Lortab), and codeine. Others include dextropropoxyphene (Darvon and Darvocet-N) and hydromorphone (Dilaudid).

Obviously, addicts who suffer from chronic pain might choose opioids as their drugs of choice because the drugs have the side benefit of pain relief.

Morphine is also an opioid. And so is heroin, which is typically synthesized from morphine. Fentanyl is another synthetic opioid, which can be 30 to 50 times more potent than heroin.

Over the last few decades, opioid prescriptions have skyrocketed in the United States, and opioid addiction has as well (with overdose deaths more than tripling between 2000 and 2016).

Unfortunately, many prescription opioid addicts eventually take up using heroin instead because in many places heroin is cheaper and easier to find. And since heroin is itself an opioid, the effect is often similar.

Of course, heroin use is far riskier. Because heroin isn't made in licensed labs under tight regulation, it's impossible for users to know the exact potency of the drug, leading to the risk of overdose. The risk of overdose has greatly increased lately now that some heroin available on the street is being laced with fentanyl.

Fentanyl is easy and cheap to produce, which makes it popular in the illegal drug trade. Some "prescription" opioid pills that are being sold by drug dealers are in fact copycat pills that actually contain fentanyl rather than a prescription painkiller. And some dealers have begun selling more exotic synthetic opioids as well, such as U-47700—in part because many obscure synthetic opioids aren't technically illegal.

Recently, there has been a spike in overdoses caused by carfentanil, an extremely potent opioid sometimes used as an elephant tranquilizer. Carfentanil can be 10,000 times as powerful as morphine. Even tiny amounts of the drug can be deadly to humans, so drug users almost never seek it out, but some dealers cut it with heroin as a cheap substitute. Because the drug can be accidentally inhaled or absorbed through the skin, police and medical personnel can be in significant danger themselves when they respond to an overdose.

The illicit opioid market is evolving rapidly, and new substances and variants are being developed all the time.

HALLUCINOGENS

Hallucinogens include LSD, psilocybin, peyote, PCP, ketamine, mescaline, and nitrous oxide. While these drugs can be dangerous in themselves, they don't generally result in addiction, although there is some evidence that people can become addicted to ketamine and PCP.

MDMA, commonly known as ecstasy or Molly, has properties of both a stimulant and a hallucinogen.

ALCOHOL

While alcohol is usually thought of as a depressant, it's a little harder to classify. Alcohol targets the same part of the brain (called GABA receptors) as classic depressant drugs. However, it can also increase norepinephrine, which is associated with stimulants.

There's some evidence that as one's blood alcohol level is rising, alcohol has a stimulant effect, but when it's falling, it has a depressant effect. This might explain why people often feel aroused and excited when they first start drinking, but later on feel fatigued and fuzzy.

MARIJUANA

Marijuana is also difficult to classify within one of the main drug families. Its principal active ingredient, called tetrahydrocannabinol or THC, works primarily by interfering with the system by which the brain's nerve cells communicate with one another.

Nerve cells typically communicate across synapses by sending neurotransmitter chemicals to receptors in the neighboring cell. In many parts of the brain, there's also an endocannabinoid system, whereby the receiving cell sends a message back to the transmitting cell, essentially providing feedback and fine-tuning how further communication should be sent. THC temporarily interferes with this feedback system, which makes communication among parts of the brain more difficult.

When communication within the brain is diminished, the results can include altered judgment, trouble with short-term memory, slower reaction times, increased appetite, impaired coordination, distorted time perception, and sometimes paranoia. The same process can also cause decreased pain sensitivity and a reduced susceptibility to nausea, which are the main reasons the drug is sometimes prescribed in a medical context.

7

What About Gambling Addiction, Sex Addiction, Etc.?

Everyone is familiar with alcoholism and drug addiction, but in recent years many people have begun describing individuals as gambling addicts, sex addicts, shopaholics, and so on. Are these real addictions, or are they just casual ways of talking about people who have bad habits?

That's a controversial question. Not everyone agrees, but the trend among professionals is toward accepting certain problematic and compulsive behaviors as addictions, at least in some cases.

The general term for addictions that don't involve substance abuse is "behavioral addictions" or "process addictions." People have claimed that such addictions can include gambling, sex, pornography, video games, Internet use, shopping, overeating, exercise, tanning, and work (hence the term "workaholic").

On the outside, these problems have a lot of the same features as substance addictions. People become obsessed with an activity and engage in it as often as possible, even when doing so has obvious destructive effects on their families, their finances, their relationships, and often their health.

The main reason that certain of these behaviors are increasingly called addictions is that studies have suggested that the repetitive activity has an effect on the brain that is similar to that of drugs—it creates a rush of dopamine that eventually alters the person's decision-making faculties. Genetic studies have also suggested that people with process addictions have genetic backgrounds similar to those of people with substance addictions.

In addition, many of the same treatments work for both. For instance, there are a number of Twelve-Step programs for behavioral addictions that have shown some success, such as Gamblers Anonymous, Overeaters Anonymous, Spenders Anonymous, and Sex Addicts Anonymous. And the drug naltrexone, which is often prescribed for both alcoholics and drug addicts, is apparently effective in treating some process addictions as well.

Finally, there appears to be a lot of cross-addiction between substance abusers and process addicts, which suggests that there is a common cause. For example, studies have found that substance abusers are 4 to 10 times more likely than the general population to have a gambling problem. (This is especially true for people who are addicted to heroin or cocaine, although we don't know exactly why.)

Most often the substance abuse happens first, but sometimes it's the other way around, and sometimes both problems start at the same time.

Some people have argued that process addictions aren't really addictions at all; they're just compulsions and might be related to obsessive–compulsive disorder. However, there are significant differences between process addictions and OCD. For instance, people who engage in process-addiction behavior tend to be trying to achieve a goal—such as winning money—and expect that they will experience pleasure as a result. On the other hand, people who have OCD might compulsively wash their hands or straighten things on their desk, but they are doing so simply to relieve tension or fear and are not expecting to enjoy the outcome.

Also, in psychological tests, people with OCD tend to score low on impulsivity and high on the desire to avoid harm to themselves, whereas people who have process addictions are often just the opposite.

In the United States, the closest thing to an impartial arbiter of addictions is the American Psychiatric Association's *DSM-5*, used for the purpose of diagnosis. *DSM-5* accepts gambling as a disorder on the same footing as substance abuse, but not any of the other process addictions.

According to the association, obsessively playing video games on the Internet *might* be such a disorder, but it requires further study. As for compulsive sex, exercise, and shopping, there's not yet enough research to establish these as bona fide mental health problems.

On the other hand, the World Health Organization, whose *ICD-10* is widely used outside the United States, has indicated that it will begin accepting "gaming disorder"—obsessively playing video games—as a problem on a par with other addictions. (*DSM-5* and *ICD-10* are discussed further in Chapter 5.)

In any event, there is considerable evidence that process addictions are functionally similar to substance addictions, at least for many people. Therefore, whenever this book refers to people who are addicted to a substance, you can assume that the same comments apply to people who have a process addiction.

There is one important difference between substance addictions and certain process addictions, however. With substance addictions, the most common goal of treatment is complete abstinence—an alcoholic shouldn't drink at all, and a heroin addict should never use heroin. However, complete abstinence obviously can't be the goal for people who are addicted to working, eating, shopping, sex, or exercise. In such cases, the goal of treatment is for addicts to simply moderate their behavior.

Interestingly, just as opioid addiction has increased in recent years, a lot of people believe that the number of people with process addictions has increased as well. There's not yet any clear statistical evidence, but there's a lot of reason to believe this is the case. For instance, certain types of process addictions, such as compulsive Internet use and video game playing, simply didn't exist more than a few decades ago. The Internet has also greatly increased the opportunity to engage in other types of process-addiction behavior. For instance, in the past, people could only gamble when they were at a casino, shop when stores were open, and work when they were at their workplace. The Internet has made it possible to engage in these activities anytime and anywhere.

II

LIVING WITH
AN ADDICT

8

How Addicts Behave

M any family members who live with an addict would probably joke that this chapter could consist of a single word: *Badly*.

But it's useful to discuss at some length how addicts behave and why. In particular, it's helpful to distinguish between three different components of addictive behavior: (1) behavior that's caused by the substance itself, (2) behavior that's caused by withdrawal, and (3) long-term personality changes caused by the effect of addiction on the brain.

Family members often don't particularly distinguish between these behaviors. They just know that the addict has changed, and not for the better.

However, being conscious of the differences can help people interact more successfully with an addict. It's also very useful to understand the differences when an addict goes into treatment, because you can expect some of the behaviors to stop immediately, a few to get worse before they get better, and some to get better but only gradually over an extended period of time. Being prepared for this can help family and friends be supportive and have realistic expectations.

BEHAVIORS CAUSED BY THE SUBSTANCE ITSELF

This type of behavior is the most variable. While the addiction process in the brain tends to be very similar for all addictive substances and behaviors, the substances have different secondary effects.

With a process addiction, it's usually very simple: The addict goes to a casino, runs up huge bills at a mall, obsessively watches pornography, and so on.

But different drugs have different properties—stimulants and depressants can cause opposite types of behavior, for example. Stimulants often make people energetic and confident, while depressants can make them drowsy and quiet. Small doses of opioids can make people more talkative, while larger doses can induce sleepiness and euphoria. Marijuana often makes people confused, relaxed, and unmotivated. (More information about the effects of different types of drugs can be found in Chapter 6.)

Alcohol is the most widely abused substance and produces the widest range of behaviors. Some alcoholics like to drink in bars around people; others go into a private room and shut the door. Alcohol makes some people withdrawn, while others can become highly emotional, angry, or even violent.

Behaviors caused by a drug tend to wear off as soon as the drug does. Addicts often have trouble remembering things that happened to them while they were drunk or high. For this reason, it's generally useless to try to communicate or interact with them while they're under the influence. (Family members of alcoholics in particular are often most tempted to complain to them about their behavior when they're drunk, and yet, in general, this is the *least* useful time to try to communicate with them.)

BEHAVIORS CAUSED BY WITHDRAWAL

When addicts aren't high on a substance, they're likely to be experiencing at least a minor form of withdrawal. The most common behavioral symptoms of withdrawal are anxiety, irritability, having difficulty concentrating, and depression. There may be physical symptoms as well, including insomnia, nausea, and sweating.

Withdrawal can be severe and unpleasant, both for addicts and for those around them. Many people who live with opioid addicts have commented that, ironically, life isn't so bad when the addict is actually using drugs. The arguments, fights, and nastiness only start when the addict is *not* currently under the influence.

The thing to remember about withdrawal is that the most severe symptoms are temporary. As an addict goes into treatment, these tend to disappear after a few days or weeks, depending on the substance and how long the person has been using it.

But that said, less extreme forms of anxiety, irritability, and depression can persist for a long time in recovery. The addict's body has developed a physiological craving, and even many months later the addict can still be experiencing its effects. This is often referred to as post-acute withdrawal syndrome.

BEHAVIORS CAUSED BY CHANGES IN THE BRAIN

Over time, addiction causes changes in the way the brain works, and these changes result in a wide variety of behavioral symptoms that are separate and apart from the behaviors that are caused directly by the drug itself or by withdrawal.

Addiction doesn't happen overnight, and these symptoms won't go away overnight, either. The immediate effects of the drug usually wear off when the drug does, and the worst symptoms of withdrawal may get better fairly quickly, but the brain changes wrought by the addiction process are more structural, and healing them can take a long time.

That's not to say that some of these symptoms can't improve quickly once an addict gets help. Many of them do. But addiction can leave a lot of scars, and it can take an addict many months or years to relearn how to interact in the world in a fully healthy way. Difficult as it may be, family members who want to be supportive in recovery will need to take this fact into account.

Behaviors that frequently accompany addiction, but that aren't caused directly by a substance, include:

Denial

Many addicts are in denial, meaning that they don't consciously recognize and take responsibility for the fact that they have a problem and that their addiction is harming them and others as well.

In part, this is because addicts often don't feel that they have done anything "wrong." And that's largely true, in the sense that they never made a deliberate choice in the beginning to hurt anyone.

But once their dependence kicks in, addicts often develop and maintain an enormous blind spot about the problem and its consequences.

This is due to their brain's having been rewired to seek the effects of the addictive substance or behavior at all costs—and the fact that consciously recognizing the downsides of their actions would interfere with this goal.

Addicts who are in denial generally perceive themselves as merely social drinkers or recreational drug users. Even heroin addicts may simply think of their drug use as "cool." They don't believe their behavior is problematic, they don't think other people should be bothered by it, and they believe that they could stop or moderate their use if they ever wanted to—they just don't see any good reason to do so.

When confronted by others about their substance use, addicts will typically brush the comment off or reassure the person that they have the situation under control and could stop anytime they wanted. If they did something egregious, they may apologize and promise to do better next time. They often actually believe that they *will* do better next time—but, of course, that's extremely unlikely.

Unfortunately, some forms of denial may persist even after the addict has been in recovery for a while. Addicts may continue to believe at some level that they didn't "really" have a problem. This can be a significant factor in causing relapse.

Defensiveness

As the disease gets worse, addicts may have a harder time shrugging off the problem or denying it to themselves. They have to go to greater and greater lengths not to consciously recognize what is happening, so that they can continue to satisfy their cravings. As their behavior becomes more clearly problematic, they may become defensive about it.

Defensiveness often takes the form of blaming others. For instance, some alcoholics may claim that they drink only because of their job, their financial circumstances, or some other life situation. If a spouse, child, or parent confronts them, they may blame the person for the problem, arguing that they drink because the spouse is inadequate in some way, the children are a disappointment, or the parent is oppressive and unfair.

Another form of defensiveness is deflection. Many addicts are brilliant in their ability to change the subject and cause a conversation to go off the rails. For instance, a wife may complain that the couple can't go out with friends anymore because the husband gets too drunk. The husband will counter by arguing that the wife spends too much money (or some other unrelated complaint). If the wife "takes the bait" and responds to the spending comment, the argument moves in a different direction and the husband has achieved his goal, which is to deflect the topic from his drinking. If the wife tries to get the subject back to the drinking, the husband will bring up something else. Or the husband might bring up a time when the couple went out without incident, which is still a way of not addressing the larger issue.

Over time, family members generally come to know one another's "hot buttons"—the things that make them upset or trigger their insecurities. For instance, a husband might be sensitive about the fact that he failed to get a promotion or be worried about a sexual problem. If he tries to confront his wife about her drinking, she might counter by blaming her problem on the fact that he's a poor earner or an inadequate lover. She knows that these are the things that are most likely to get him upset and move the conversation off to a different subject. This is also her way of "punishing" him for bringing up her drinking and trying to discourage him from doing it again.

Defensiveness is an area where a symptom of the addiction is often confused with the effect of the substance itself. For instance, an alcoholic might come home drunk and deliberately start an argument. Many people would assume that he's arguing because he's drunk—that the behavior is caused by the alcohol. In fact, though, the alcoholic might come home drunk and anticipate being criticized. To prevent this, he proactively picks an argument on a different topic. The arguing happens not only because he's drunk, but also because he's defensive.

Irresponsibility

As addiction gets worse, addicts have less and less ability to handle the ordinary responsibilities of everyday life. They may do poorly at work or get fired. They may neglect household chores or parental responsibilities. They may forget to pay bills, maintain their car, or do their taxes.

It's important to note that when an addict first goes into treatment, this problem doesn't magically disappear. When an addict is first getting well, it often takes every bit of concentration he or she can muster just to remain clean and sober. The ability to handle a full plate of life responsibilities in addition to maintaining sobriety is something that may only come back to the person over an extended period of time.

Immaturity

Because addicts' ordinary mental processes are overwhelmed by an imperative to seek a drug, and because they're often working hard not to be fully conscious of their situation, they're very likely to make poor life decisions. They may be adults, but they behave in many ways like children because the rational adult functioning of their brain has been significantly impaired.

Immature behavior can include getting into fights, driving while drunk or high, quitting a job for no good reason, sexual promiscuity, getting into inappropriate relationships, failing to make or stick to a budget, engaging in risky activities, and generally making choices without considering the consequences.

This can particularly be a problem for young people, who don't have a lot of the maturity that comes from experience to begin with.

It's often said that the brain does not mature during the time one has an addiction. Thus, if a person develops an addiction at age 16 and eventually gets into recovery at age 25, he or she may have a "maturity gap" spanning those years. Many parents in situations like this have observed that even though their children are in their mid-20s and are now in successful long-term recovery, they continue to make immature life choices more consistent with those of a 16-year-old.

The good news is that young people in these circumstances are typically able to "catch up" emotionally. There's not a lot of scientific research on this point, but therapists generally believe that the recovering brain is eventually able to heal the maturity gap, although it can take some time.

Isolation

When addiction hijacks the brain's pleasure center, it causes the addict to gradually lose the ability to experience pleasure from any source other than substance abuse. For this reason, addicts gradually cease to enjoy social activities and other people's company. Worse, they may experience other people as a threat because other people might bring up their troubling behavior or try to get them to stop.

For this reason, as the disease progresses, addicts tend to isolate themselves. If they spend time with anyone, it will commonly be with other addicts who are unlikely to be critical.

In addition, addicts' defensiveness often alienates friends and loved ones. So not only do addicts not want to spend time with other people, but other people often don't want to spend time with them.

Of course, this is a vicious circle: Addicts become estranged from the very people who might be able to support and help them.

In recovery, addicts often have to learn how to become social again. For instance, family members may still harbor a great deal of anger, and it will be necessary to mend relationships, rebuild bridges, and restore trust. This can take a lot of effort and time.

Often, an addict has lost a great many friendships and social contacts. And many addicts don't want to renew their old friendships, either because of shame or because the old friends may trigger their addictive tendencies—the last thing a recovering alcoholic needs is to renew acquaintances with former drinking buddies, for example.

As a result, many recovering addicts have to start all over again socially. This can actually be one of the chief advantages of support groups such as Alcoholics Anonymous—they give recovering addicts a chance to meet new people who are likely to understand their situation and not be judgmental.

Self-Centeredness

As the brain becomes overwhelmed by the need to satisfy an addictive craving, and substance abuse becomes addicts' only source of pleasure—and in the end the only thing they can really think about—they are likely to become selfish and self-centered in the literal sense of the term. Like a panicked drowning person, they are trying to save themselves and can't stop to think about others.

Of course, this can be maddening for families. Family members may go to enormous lengths to try to help an addict, and the addict never thinks of doing anything for them in return.

As with irresponsibility, it's important to note that in recovery this problem doesn't disappear right away. Especially at the beginning, it can take every bit of a recovering addict's effort just to stay clean and sober. The ability to genuinely consider other people's needs and feelings usually comes back slowly over time.

Manipulation

In the later stages of the disease, as addicts become desperate, they can also become highly manipulative. Their only thought is of getting a substance, and they become willing to take advantage of people—even people they love—for this purpose.

At this stage, addicts lie. Addicts steal. Addicts ask for money for food and spend it on gambling. Addicts borrow a car to go to an AA meeting and go to a liquor store instead. Addicts excuse themselves to go to the bathroom and instead rifle through their mother's purse looking for cash.

Addicts can make up elaborate stories to fool their loved ones to get what they need to satisfy their cravings. More than one family member has commented that the addict in their life was deserving of an Academy Award. "I can't believe I fell for it," they say. Addicts can act and pretend and dissemble as though their life depended on it—because, in their mind, it does.

A FINAL THOUGHT

In considering this list of behaviors triggered by the addiction process, it's easy to see why so many people have for so long thought of addiction as a moral fault. A lot of the behaviors—irresponsibility, self-centeredness, manipulation, and so forth—actually *are* moral faults when considered in isolation and when they're not caused by a brain disorder. So it's not hard to understand why loved ones often find it so difficult not to be angry and feel betrayed and to continue to love the addict while hating the disease.

Of course, addicts also tend to blame themselves morally at some deep level and to feel tremendous shame and guilt about their behavior. These feelings of shame and guilt are often a big part of the reason that addicts are reluctant to admit their problem and seek help. And sadly, once addicts go into recovery and start reflecting on their life, their shame and guilt may increase—which can make them more likely to relapse.

9

How Loved Ones
Are Affected

Addiction is a family disease. When an addict gets sick, it's not just the addict who gets sick. The entire family is affected in a profound way.

Families are a system. Over time, family members come to understand one another very deeply and to have ingrained ways of doing things, from dividing labor to having fun together. They know how to love and support one another and how to ask for and receive love and support. They know one another's personalities and what to expect from one another.

Addiction destroys this system. When one person's behavior and personality start to change dramatically for no apparent reason, everyone's world is thrown into turmoil.

And the changes are not for the better. Family members who used to rely on the addict for everything from income to emotional support to chores around the house now have to deal with someone who may be erratic, self-centered, argumentative, unreliable, and distant, not to mention a source of constant drama and anxiety.

Addiction has broken up a lot of homes. Many spouses have filed for divorce. Children have completely walked away from their families—or been kicked out of the house. Couples who have a child who is an addict have split up simply because of the difficulty of the experience, especially if they can't agree with each other on how to handle the situation.

There are two important points here. One is that every member of an addict's household is profoundly harmed by what they go through. They may handle it in different ways, but they are all hurt, and they all need help.

The second point is that this is *normal*. Because there's a stigma to addiction and many people are secretive about it, a lot of families believe that their experience is unique and that no one else can understand it. But in fact, the tremendous familial upset caused by addiction is all too common. Indeed, it's hard to imagine a family reacting in any other way.

Here are some of the emotions and reactions that family members *typically* have when dealing with an addict:

CONFUSION AND UNCERTAINTY

When family members first begin to suspect that someone is an addict—when their life first starts to be disrupted—there can be a great deal of confusion and uncertainty.

Sometimes addicts are very good at hiding their consumption. In such cases, what the family first notices are personality and behavioral changes. The person may become more irritable, short-tempered, lazy, distant, or defensive. The addict may stay out late, sleep late, or disappear. Only later does the family realize that a substance is causing the problem.

In other cases, the family is aware that the person is drinking more than usual or using drugs but is reluctant to conclude that he or she is an addict. Although addiction affects people in every walk of life, many family members want to believe that their loved one is "not that sort of person." Addiction is scary, and many people resist coming to the conclusion that it's affecting someone they love. Besides, addiction is not like most illnesses, where you can go to a doctor and get a test to tell you whether you have it or not. As a result, many people remain confused and uncertain for a long time as to whether their loved one is in fact addicted to something.

SELF-DOUBT

Closely related to confusion and uncertainty is self-doubt. Even if it's so obvious that an addict has a problem that family members can no longer reasonably be uncertain about it, they will sometimes doubt their own understanding of what's going on. This is usually the result of the addict's behavior—denying, deflecting, crafting excuses, outright lying, and doing everything possible to undermine other family members' perceptions.

Self-doubt is different from being in denial. It's not an outright refusal to admit the problem in order to avoid the psychological pain that would result. Rather, it's the consequence of being constantly lied to by someone you used to be able to trust.

A term some people use to describe this phenomenon is "gaslighting," after the 1944 Ingrid Bergman film *Gaslight*, in which a husband constantly deceives his wife to make her believe she is losing her mind. Of course, addicts aren't deliberately scheming to make family members question their sanity; they're just trying to get the criticism to stop. But the effect of the continual lying is similar—family members often end up repeatedly second-guessing their own understanding of what's happening around them.

STRESS

Addiction is stressful for everyone in the family. The fact that the family dynamic has been disrupted is highly stressful in itself, as everyone has to cope with the changes. In addition, there can be tremendous worry and anxiety about what will happen to the person and what to do next. Plus, the addict's behavior itself tends to raise the stress level. The addict may act irresponsibly, pick fights, argue, break promises, spill or break things, make noise late at night, and so on. Living with an alcoholic in particular can often be comparable to having a toddler in the house.

Many people adapt to the addict's behavior by treading carefully and trying not to trigger an argument. But this constant attempt to avoid the stress of a confrontation also produces a great deal of stress in and of itself.

ANGER

Families of addicts are often furious. They are mad about the changes in their life and mad that the addict is behaving in an irresponsible way.

Also, addicts who become irritable or defensive often say things to family members that are deeply cruel and cutting and can send those family members into a rage.

Unfortunately, anger begets anger. When family members vent their fury at the addict, the addict typically responds in kind, and shouting matches can become a regular part of the landscape.

In the heat of the moment, when an addict is being obnoxious, it's very difficult to remember that the person has a disease—especially since addicts who want to deflect blame usually know exactly how to push someone's buttons to get a reaction. At that point, it's hard for family members to feel anything other than that the addict is simply a jerk.

EMOTIONAL HURT

A good deal of the anger that family members feel is caused by emotional pain—the sense that the addict has betrayed them, has rejected them, and doesn't love them anymore.

It's easy to see why family members feel this way. The addict is *behaving* as though he doesn't love them. He doesn't do anything nice for them, doesn't listen to them, and refuses to change his actions so as to spare them pain.

Families of addicts generally cry—a lot. It can feel as though someone you deeply love and trust has simply broken up with you and walked off, without even providing the solace of an explanation.

MISTRUST

Because addicts become adept at lying and manipulating, family members often stop trusting them. They usually *want* to trust them—to believe them when they make excuses, promise to do better, and so on—but they have been disappointed so many times that it becomes difficult if not impossible to do so.

Family members frequently feel bad about their own mistrust, not only because it's sad not to be able to have confidence in a loved one, but because they feel they *should* trust the person—that it's somehow wrong not to think the best of someone they care deeply about.

However, it's important to remember that trust is not a gift that you can simply choose to give; it has to be earned. It's built up over time like a wall, brick by brick, through many small actions of telling the truth and keeping one's word. Addiction knocks down the wall. And family members can't simply repair the wall even if they want to; recovering addicts have to do that themselves through repeatedly demonstrating that they are once again worthy of trust.

GUILT

Family members often feel guilt. Lacking any other explanation for the addict's actions, they think that perhaps they are somehow at fault and that they did something wrong. Of course, addicts often play on and encourage these feelings because doing so deflects blame from themselves and enables them to avoid confronting the truth.

Parents of teenage and young adult addicts are especially prone to feeling guilt. All parents tend to worry about whether they did a good enough job raising their children, and it's intensely painful to see a child head down such a self-destructive path. In addition, parents are often friends with people who have children of similar ages. No matter how supportive these friends may try to be, if they haven't experienced a similar problem, they may subconsciously communicate the idea that the parents are somehow responsible.

Young children of addicts are also particularly vulnerable to feeling guilt, and it cannot be emphasized strongly enough to them that what they are experiencing is not their fault and that they didn't cause their parent's addiction.

Guilt is often the result of simply not being able to find any other explanation for a loved one's actions. When someone we love begins acting very negatively, and we can't figure out why, it's a very stressful experience. Feeling guilty—assigning blame to oneself—can be very uncomfortable, but it can actually be a lot less uncomfortable than living with the inability to come up with any explanation at all. And addiction, of course, is an incredibly baffling condition. That's another reason it's so important to understand that addiction is a specific chemical process in the brain. This understanding can help families move beyond guilt and blame and toward taking constructive action to get help for a loved one.

OBSESSION

After a while, it often seems that the only thing that family members of an addict ever think about is the addict.

They worry constantly about the person and about what the person's behavior is doing to the family. They try to understand what is happening and why the addict's actions don't seem to make any sense. They think a great deal about their confrontations with the addict or make enormous efforts to avoid confrontations. Eventually, thoughts about the addict tend to crowd out everything else in the family members' lives and disrupt their work, school, friendships, leisure, exercise habits, and overall health. In other words, just as addiction takes over the addict's whole life, it eventually takes over the family's whole life as well.

Sadly, the obsessional patterns may not get any better—and may in fact grow worse—when the addict makes an effort at recovery. When an addict is first trying not to use, the family may worry intensely every time the person is alone. Even an addict's simply going off briefly to use the bathroom can trigger alarm bells. The family may worry about whether the addict is going to enough meetings, or taking therapy seriously enough, or following all the other steps necessary to avoid a relapse, even as the addict appears blithely unconcerned about these issues. It's not at all uncommon for families of addicts to exclaim, "I'm working harder at their recovery than they are!"

ISOLATION

Families of addicts often cut themselves off from friends, relatives, and normal social and recreational activities.

Because addiction is so often a source of shame and embarrassment, and because addicts' behavior can be so unpredictable, families often stop inviting people to their home for fear that visitors will discover the "family secret." Children who are normally outgoing can become socially withdrawn because it's awkward for them to spend time at friends' houses and then be unable to reciprocate—or even explain why they can't.

Couples routinely stop going out with friends when one of them becomes an addict. In fact, they often stop going out at all because of the likelihood that an evening out will devolve into a "scene."

Even if friends and relatives know about the addiction, this may not help. Many people will stop spending time with an addict's family because they feel awkward about the "elephant in the room" and don't know what to say. And sometimes friends and relatives will react by being so hostile, preachy, or full of bad advice that the family members themselves decide to spend less time around them.

On top of this, family members commonly decline social or recreational opportunities simply because they're too busy worrying about the addict or responding to his or her behavior—which only deepens the isolation.

INADEQUACY

Family members often derive a great deal of satisfaction from being able to play a particular role within the family. For instance, one family member might play the role of the provider or protector, the one who acts as the breadwinner or keeps the family safe. Another might play a nurturing role and make others feel loved, comforted, and secure. A parent or grandparent might take satisfaction in being able to provide support, guidance, and help to a child, and a child might take satisfaction in being able to bring joy and laughter to a parent.

When someone in a family develops an addiction, the ability of other family members to play these roles is often severely disrupted. An addict's spouse may feel completely unable to protect, nurture, or comfort the person or to keep him or her safe from the consequences of the addiction. A parent may feel unable to protect or offer guidance to an addicted child, and a child may feel unable to please (or appease) an addicted parent.

This takes an emotional toll on the family members. A key source of their sense of self-worth has been taken away, and they are often left bewildered by their inability to play a role that gave them such pride and satisfaction. Their powerlessness to solve or even respond effectively to the person's addiction can leave them with a debilitating sense of inadequacy.

GRIEF

Grief is the process of mourning a loss, such as a loved one's passing away. But grief doesn't have to involve a literal death. Even if an addict is very much alive, family members often grieve a loss—the loss of the person the addict once was and the loss of the relationship they once had with him or her.

Everyone grieves differently, and there is no one "right" way to grieve, but it's not uncommon for people who have experienced a profound loss to feel depressed. A certain amount of depression can be an entirely normal reaction to losing a relationship with a loved one. Of course, anyone experiencing a severe or debilitating depression should see a therapist for help. And it's a good idea in general for family members of an addict to discuss how the problem has affected their own lives with a therapist, preferably one who has experience and training in the addiction field.

In fact, if you put all these typical family reactions together—anger, stress, guilt, hurt, and so on—you can see why it's not uncommon for families to descend into despair and even desperation. Addiction is a family disease because it doesn't just make addicts dysfunctional; it makes entire families dysfunctional.

Of course, addicts can get well, and families can also get well. But just as addicts usually need treatment, families may also need various kinds of help. Therapy and support groups can provide tremendous relief to family members. So can taking the time to care for themselves through relaxation activities, exercise, proper diet, getting enough sleep, and so on.

It often seems impossible to do these things, particularly when family members are caught up in obsessing about the addict: "How can I go to the movies when I need to be worrying?" This is why it's important to remember that the addict is not the only person in the family who is sick and not the only person who needs to be cared for. Addicts may be the most dramatic and attention-grabbing victims, but they're not the only ones.

• • • • • • • • 10 • • • • • • •

Denial, Enabling,
and Codependency

As discussed in the previous chapter, families can be thought of as systems. Family members adapt to one another and adjust their behavior around the other members' behavior. When everyone is adapting successfully, the family functions well and everything feels "normal."

When a family member develops an addiction, however, the system is thrown completely out of whack. All of a sudden one person has changed and created a lot of problems. Very frequently, other family members find ways over time to adapt to addicts' behavior. They "walk on eggshells" around them so as not to "set them off." They make excuses for their actions to friends and relatives. They cover for them if they miss work or other obligations. They pick up the slack at home when they ignore family responsibilities. And so on.

Typically, this doesn't happen all at once. It's a gradual process. Little by little, the family adjusts, and living with the addict's behavior eventually becomes "the new normal."

The problem is that this "new normal" isn't normal at all. It's highly dysfunctional. It's often extremely stressful and can cause enormous mental, emotional, and even physical problems for family members.

When trying to describe this sort of unhealthy adaptation, three terms that are commonly used are *denial, enabling,* and *codependency.* For better or worse, these terms have become part of the lexicon of pop psychology, which means that well-meaning friends and relatives often use them without really understanding them. This chapter discusses these concepts in detail because understanding what they actually mean can help a family move from a dysfunctional "normality" to a healthier way of coping.

DENIAL

Both addicts and their families can be in denial. But there's a difference between the two.

In the addict's brain, the prefrontal cortex is overwhelmed and partially disabled by the dopamine-related changes. As a result, the addict cannot make rational observations or decisions about substance use and often literally cannot perceive how much of a problem the use of substances is causing. The addiction process itself prevents the person from understanding that he or she has a problem. This is a *biological* form of denial.

There can also be a *psychological* form of denial. This is a defense mechanism in which the psyche deals with a terrible event or piece of news—one that would otherwise cause trauma—by simply not recognizing or processing it. Both addicts and their families can have this type of denial, since it is often very difficult for people to accept that they or someone they love has a serious problem such as addiction.

It's important to note that psychological denial is not an illness, and a certain amount of it can be completely normal. Denial exists to protect us from experiences that would otherwise be a terrible shock to our mental and emotional well-being. It allows us to come to terms with traumatic experiences in a gradual way rather than in a sudden and debilitating way. For instance, in her book *On Death and Dying*, Elisabeth Kübler-Ross suggested that people who are diagnosed with a terminal illness often experience some form of denial, and this can be a natural part of the process of coming to terms with such a devastating piece of news.

It's also important to note that denial is different from uncertainty. Many people suspect that a family member may be an addict, but they are reluctant to come to this conclusion and want to give the person the benefit of the doubt. They don't want to accept that the person is an addict unless the evidence is unmistakably clear. This is not denial. It's only denial if someone refuses to believe that a person is an addict *even though* the evidence is unmistakably clear.

It's a common situation for one family member to be in denial about someone's addiction while others are not. This usually leads to extended arguments between the family members, which are debilitating to everyone involved and not particularly helpful in getting the addict into treatment.

The truth is that denial is not necessarily harmful to the family member who is in denial. Remember, denial is a defense mechanism; the person wouldn't be in denial unless, *in his or her mind*, the alternative was psychologically unbearable. The real problem is that the person's being in denial may be harmful to the addict. Addicts are very frequently in denial themselves, and having a family member who is also in denial makes it easier for them to continue to not recognize their problem and to engage in addictive behavior. A family member's being in denial allows the disease to progress and the addict to avoid treatment.

Most people who are dealing with a family member who is in denial try to reason the person out of it with logic. ("But Mom, he *must* be an addict. Look at what happened last week.") The problem with this approach is that denial is a psychological defense mechanism—it has nothing to do with logic, and a person cannot be reasoned out of it because it's not based on reason in the first place.

A better approach is to understand that denial is based on fear. A person who is in denial about a family member's addiction is terrified about the problem and has set up a psychological wall against that terror. So the best strategy may be to reduce the fear. This could be done by demystifying addiction—providing information about how it's not a moral failing, what happens in the brain, the different treatment options, how treatment can often be successful, how people in all walks of life are susceptible to addiction, and so on. Making addiction seem less traumatic may cause people to lower their defenses.

Ideally, this should be done in a nonthreatening way, because "hitting someone over the head" with information is likely only to further trigger the defense mechanism.

Denial and Legal Substances

Because addiction affects the brain in fundamentally the same way regardless of the addict's drug of choice, addicts tend to be equally in denial regardless of the substance they're using. Even intravenous heroin users somehow manage to rationalize their habit and argue that it's no big deal and that other people shouldn't be so worried about it.

However, there's no question that addicts and family members have an easier time remaining in denial about substance abuse if the substance being abused is legal. For instance, an alcoholic might point out that other family members drink, and perhaps even that other family members occasionally drink to excess. While these facts are irrelevant to the question of whether the person is an alcoholic, they can sometimes make it harder for family and friends to stand their ground and insist that the person has a serious problem.

With marijuana now legalized in parts of the United States, Canada, and elsewhere, the same issue can arise.

In fact, marijuana is a particularly difficult case because many areas have legalized the drug specifically for medicinal purposes. And while marijuana arguably has some legitimate medical benefits in the case of serious illnesses such as cancer, there's no question that a number of opportunistic "weed doctors" have begun authorizing unlimited marijuana purchases by nearly anyone who comes in their door and makes vague complaints about stress, anxiety, or occasional lack of interest in sex. The result is that, when family and friends challenge a marijuana addict, the addict can often accuse them of trying to interfere with a doctor's legitimately prescribed course of medical treatment.

This is a new problem for families. Alcohol and tobacco have been legal for a long time, but no one has ever claimed to have been ordered by a physician to smoke a pack a day or get drunk every night. And while prescription painkillers are legal, no doctor ever authorizes a patient to purchase an unlimited supply.

Another problematic drug is Suboxone, which is used to treat opioid addiction in some cases. But it also has opioid properties itself and is often sold illegally and abused. Some addicts buy it on the street and claim to be in recovery and "self-medicating" with it, but in fact they're simply abusing opioids in a different way. (See Chapter 28 for more information on Suboxone.)

For family and friends, the important thing to remember is that addiction isn't justified by a prescription or by the fact that a substance can have legal or even medical uses. If a loved one claims to be using a substance for legitimate reasons but is in fact abusing it in an addictive manner, he or she is in denial.

ENABLING

Enabling is behavior that makes it easier for an addict to be an addict.

Since family members have a natural tendency to adapt to each other and to make everything "normal," it's extremely common for them, especially in the beginning, to react to an addict's behavioral problems by picking up the slack so that the family system continues to function. Unfortunately, the lessons that addicts typically learn from this pattern are that it's okay to be an addict, that there are no negative consequences to their behavior, and that no matter how irresponsible they become as a result of using, someone will be there to pick up the pieces. In this way, the efforts of family members to "help" often end up exacerbating the problem.

The best way to illustrate enabling behavior is through examples. While not true in every case, all of the following can be enabling:

- Buying alcohol for an alcoholic
- Making excuses to friends for an addict's behavior
- Dragging an addict into bed after he or she passes out
- Calling in sick for an addict
- Taking on household chores the addict used to do
- Cleaning up messes the addict made
- Bailing an addict out of legal trouble
- Giving a child money that you believe will be used for drugs
- Paying rent or other debts for a child who spent his or her own money on drugs
- Paying off a debt to a drug dealer
- Taking on an addict's personal responsibilities
- Blaming others for things that are the addict's fault
- Accepting abusive behavior

Many people confuse denial and enabling. Denial is very often a cause of enabling, of course, but they are separate things. Denial is a psychological defense mechanism; enabling is a pattern of behavior. You can have one without the other. For instance, a wife can be in denial that her husband is an alcoholic, but she can still decide that he's behaving badly and refuse to do things for him that he should do himself. That's denial but not enabling. On the other hand, a couple can be fully aware that their daughter is a drug addict but still clean up all the problems she causes in her life because they want to "help" her. That's enabling without denial.

Enabling tends to be highly stressful and dysfunctional for the enabler and to be counterproductive in terms of getting someone in active addiction to agree to treatment. Nearly all addiction professionals believe that addicts are much more likely to agree to treatment if they're forced to experience the natural consequences of their behavior rather than having someone constantly make all the negative aspects of their addiction disappear.

The problem is that stopping enabling can be very difficult to do.

All of us are wired to want to help our family members and to prevent them from being hurt. The idea of sitting back and allowing a loved one to suffer rather than stepping in and helping is very counterintuitive. It causes us pain to see a loved one in pain.

Furthermore, we generally feel guilty when we allow someone we care about to experience unpleasant consequences. And addicts are very accomplished at playing on this feeling. It's completely typical for addicts to accuse family members who refuse to enable them of not loving them, of being uncaring and heartless, or much worse.

In addition, there are limits to the kinds of natural consequences we are willing to—or should—allow. It's one thing to refuse to help a child file tax returns on time. It's another to allow a child to be put in actual physical danger. We want the addict to get well, but we don't want him or her to die or be seriously injured in the process.

Again, addicts can be highly manipulative in this regard. They don't ask for money for drugs; they say they desperately need the money for food or rent and so on.

The desire to stop enabling can sometimes put families in an extremely difficult bind, where there is no easy answer and every option seems like a bad one. For instance:

- It might be enabling to provide liquor to an alcoholic, but what if an alcoholic threatens to go to the liquor store himself, and he might drive drunk while doing so?
- It might be enabling to call in sick or otherwise make excuses for an addict at work, but what if the alternative is that she loses her job?

- It might be enabling to allow a child to continue living at home rather than going to rehab, but what if the alternative is turning the child out of the house with no place to live?
- It might be enabling to bail a child out of legal problems, but what if the alternative is that the child goes to jail or faces an impossible debt?

Many families will tell you that it took an extreme act of refusing to enable to put their loved one on the right path. For instance, they will say that their child only became serious about treatment once it became unmistakably clear to the son or daughter that the alternative was homelessness or prison. Of course, such an extreme act is emotionally gut-wrenching for all concerned. And there's never a guarantee that it won't backfire or make things even worse. Families are usually able to make such a decision only after they have tried everything else and feel that they have no other option left.

In the end, only you can decide what truly is enabling and how best to respond to any given situation. Lots of people can give advice, but you're the one who has to live with your decisions. However, it's extremely helpful to be aware of the phenomenon and to take it into account. Simply asking the question "Am I enabling?" before doing something for an addict can go a long way toward making a family situation less dysfunctional.

By the way, some people don't like the term "enabling" and prefer to say "protecting behaviors." The reason is that it's never the *intent* of the family to enable the addiction; their intent is to protect the addict from harm. The problem, of course, is that such behaviors usually also end up protecting the addiction from being properly treated.

CODEPENDENCY

Codependency describes a relationship in which one partner makes great sacrifices to help (or, very commonly, to enable) the other partner who suffers from an addiction or similar problem. A codependent person is usually described as someone who is needy, has low self-esteem, is excessively attached to the addicted partner, and frequently behaves as a martyr. It's a codependency because each person is emotionally dependent on the other.

The term "codependency" was initially used to describe romantic relationships, but lately it has been applied more broadly to include other types of family members or friends.

A lot of people confuse enabling and codependency, but they are very different. Enabling is a kind of behavior that anyone can easily fall into. Almost all families of addicts engage in some form of enabling when the problem first appears; they generally stop only when they learn from painful experience that it only makes the problem worse. A codependent person, on the other hand, doesn't engage in enabling-type behavior out of a misplaced desire to help the addict; rather, codependent people do so to fulfill their own psychological needs and will continue to do so even if they become aware that it won't help the addict recover.

"Codependent" is a popular term for a certain type of personality. It's not a formal psychological disorder of the sort recognized by the American Psychiatric Association in its *DSM-5*, for instance, and as a result, most psychologists will not diagnose or treat it. (*DSM-5* does include something called "dependent personality disorder," but that refers to people who rely excessively on others for advice and direction in life in general and isn't limited to relationships with addicts.)

The idea of codependency arose initially within Alcoholics Anonymous. It was popularized in the 1980s by books such as *Women Who Love Too Much* by Robin Norwood and *Codependent No More* by Melody Beattie. There is a national support group, based on AA, called Co-Dependents Anonymous.

The term "codependency" is used a great deal, but it's a good idea to be careful with it. Codependency generally refers to a personality tendency that would exist *regardless* of whether the person was currently involved with an addict. Many people who try to diagnose themselves or others with codependency are in reality just describing the natural responses of an individual to the difficult situation of living with someone with an addiction and the sort of obsessing and enabling that everyone is prone to before realizing that it doesn't help.

In fact, an interesting study by a Stanford University professor found that among a high percentage of people who appeared to have the characteristics of codependency, the symptoms disappeared once the person's partner went into recovery and the person no longer had to live with someone who was actively drinking or using drugs.

11

The Stigma of Addiction

There's no question that addiction is stigmatized in our society. Addicts are often ashamed to admit to their problem, and so are their families. Addicts face conscious or unconscious discrimination in employment, insurance, health care, government benefits, and many other aspects of life. Friends and relatives may forever shun people who have an addiction, or at least look at them suspiciously and trust them less. And simply admitting to an addiction can have serious criminal consequences.

A great deal could be written about the social and public policy need to remove this stigma (including the fact that the stigma results in more limited funds for research and treatment compared to other illnesses), but that's beyond the scope of this book. This chapter will discuss the ways in which the stigma affects addicts and their families on a personal level.

HOW THE STIGMA AFFECTS PEOPLE

Encouraging Denial

The first way that the stigma affects people is that it encourages denial. Remember, denial is a psychological defense mechanism triggered by the psyche's need to keep at bay something it experiences as scary or traumatic. The fact that a person has an addiction is terrible enough, but the fact that it might also lead to a lifetime of discrimination, suspicion, and treatment as a second-class citizen makes acknowledging it even harder to accept. As a result, both addicts and their family members are more likely to deny the reality for as long as possible.

Feeding Shame

Closely related to denial is shame. Addicts often feel tremendous shame about the fact that they can't just "get ahold of themselves" and stop using. This shame is almost entirely the result of a society that tells addicts that they are inferior people who lack willpower and are moral failures. Addicts typically also feel shame about the way in which they have treated the people they love as a result of their problems.

Shame doesn't just feed denial; it also leads to feelings of anxiety, depression, low self-esteem, and worthlessness. And as we've seen, very often the reason addicts start using substances in the first place is to combat precisely those feelings. Thus, the stigma produces a vicious circle in which an addict abuses substances to avoid feelings of anxiety and depression, but doing so only ends up intensifying those very feelings and encouraging more abuse.

Family members also feel shame. Because the disease is so stigmatized, family members may have a hard time admitting and confronting their own feelings and may instead lash out at the addict or at one another. Parents of addicted children are especially prone to feeling shame because they may assume that they're somehow at fault for their child's problems or because friends, relatives, and others may *think* that they're at fault.

Promoting Silence

Another way in which the stigma harms people is that it encourages silence. Even addicts and families who are not in denial about the problem often never speak about it to anyone else and go to considerable lengths to cover it up. It becomes the family secret. (If you think about it, even the fact that the leading support group for alcoholics has the word "Anonymous" in its title suggests that members shouldn't want to reveal their names because their condition is something shameful.)

Silence separates people from help. It makes addicts reluctant to go to therapy or to support groups because they're afraid they will have to "confess their sins." And it makes it hard for family members to talk about their problems with friends and get the kind of social support they would normally receive for all sorts of other life problems.

"Family secrets," by the way, are a classic symptom of dysfunctional families where people's negative adaptations produce stress and unhappiness.

Harming Relationships

The stigma of addiction also warps relations with relatives and friends who are told (or who otherwise find out) about the addict's situation. Few people are able to treat someone the same once they know that the person has a history of addiction. As for the addict's family members, they often find that relatives and friends who know about the problem will bombard them with all sorts of suggestions and advice that are unhelpful at best and downright offensive at worst. This bad advice is generally due to ignorance of the real nature of the problem—which is in turn due to the stigma.

Negatively Affecting Medical Care

One other way in which the stigma harms addicts has to do with the fact that even medical professionals—who should be the first in line to understand addiction—often don't make enough of an effort to comprehend the addict's situation. Sadly, while a lot of doctors and nurses will give lip service to the idea that addiction is a disease, the stigma often prevents them from taking it as seriously as they would a more traditional diagnosis or educating themselves as to how to properly handle a patient who is an addict. (An example might be a surgeon who doesn't give sufficient thought to prescribing painkillers for a patient who is in recovery.)

WHERE STIGMA COMES FROM

Addiction is stigmatized in almost every culture, although there is some variation. For instance, many countries are more tolerant of male addicts than female ones, and countries in which alcohol plays an important cultural role, such as Russia, may be more tolerant of alcoholism than, say, some predominantly Muslim countries.

It's obviously not possible to single-handedly change an entire society's attitude toward addiction, but it might be possible to change one's own attitude—or that of certain family members or friends—by reflecting on where the stigma comes from.

In a way, there's nothing special about the stigma of addiction. Societies around the world have always applied a stigma to diseases and other problems that they don't understand well. The reason is that anything harmful that we don't understand is scary, and a common reaction to fear is to push the scary thing away—to treat it as "other," and to say that the scary thing is bad and that it can't possibly affect me because I'm good. This is a form of denial, but on a society-wide scale. People stigmatize diseases they don't understand because doing so defends them psychologically against the realization that the disease could in fact affect them or someone they care about.

One way in which this happens is a widespread mistaken assumption that the disease is limited to "undesirable" populations. For instance, in the early days of the polio epidemic in the United States, it was widely believed that polio was a disease solely of the urban poor. (President Franklin Roosevelt, who had polio, was always careful to keep it a secret from voters.)

When typhus fever and cholera struck New York City in the 1890s, the diseases were widely blamed on Jewish immigrants, who were often quarantined even though they were perfectly healthy. Closer to our own day, many people continued to assume that AIDS was a disease found only among gay men even long after science showed that this was not the case.

In the same way, many people who don't want to think that addiction could happen to them or their family tend to associate it in their minds with "other" or supposedly less worthy populations and to maintain the attitude that "we're not those kinds of people."

Another aspect of disease stigma is avoidance—the reluctance to associate with someone who has the disease, or even to talk about the disease, for fear that it will somehow make it seem closer.

This can result in a mistaken belief that a disease is contagious. For instance, many people believed for years that cancer was contagious long after this was disproven, and as a result it was difficult for cancer survivors to find jobs and children were not allowed to play at a house where someone had cancer. (In fact, for many years it was common for people not to even speak the word "cancer." When someone died of cancer, obituaries would often simply say that the person had passed away "after a long illness.")

Obesity is another condition that is frequently misunderstood. As with addiction, obese people are commonly ridiculed, blamed for a lack of willpower, and shunned socially.

Seen in this way, the stigma of addiction is not so special—it's just another example of a very common but unfortunate social process of denying the reality of something that is scary and hard to understand. The best way to combat stigma is with information and learning as much as possible about the condition so that it doesn't seem so baffling and frightening. The less mysterious addiction is, the less need there will be to deny that it exists or to treat it as something to be ashamed of.

12

Strategies to Get a Loved One into Treatment

When people realize that a family member or close friend may have a substance abuse problem, their initial instinct is usually to try to talk the person out of it. "Surely I can make them see reason," they think. After all, it's obvious that it's a serious problem, and it's obvious what to do about it. (Just stop.)

When that doesn't work, family members usually resort to the rest of the arsenal of techniques that relatives use to influence one another. These can include begging, pleading, bargaining, wheedling, screaming, shaming, and inflicting guilt.

Most of the time, none of this has any effect.

The reason these approaches don't work is not that addicts are bad people, or that they don't understand how they're hurting themselves and those around them, or that they have stopped caring about their family—although family members are often tempted to think (and to say) such things.

The reason these approaches don't work is that the dopamine-related changes in the brain have hijacked the addict's decision-making process. They have impaired the person's free will.

Imagine an old-fashioned balance scale. Most of the time we decide whether to engage in an action by weighing the costs on one side and the benefits on the other. If the benefits outweigh the costs, we continue. If the costs start to outweigh the benefits, we stop.

73

Family members who are trying to talk addicts out of their behavior are attempting to add weight to the costs side of the scale. But the problem is that the scale is rigged—the addiction has unfairly added a very heavy thumb to the benefits side, so that no matter how many good arguments family members put on the costs side, the benefits side still wins.

(Of course, there are always stories of people who were simply talked out of drinking or using drugs. But in such cases, the person was almost always in reality just a heavy drinker or recreational user who had also repeatedly made poor life decisions—and not truly an addict in the physiological sense.)

So, what can be done to persuade an addict to stop using and to begin treatment?

While the changes in the brain caused by addiction *impair* an addict's free will, that doesn't mean that an addict ceases to have any free will at all. The scale still works; it just has a heavy unfair weight on the benefits side. But if a family can put enough weight on the costs side—or can adjust the way that the addict views the costs and benefits—it may be possible to get him or her to make better decisions. Addicts *will* stop if the costs begin to outweigh the benefits *in their mind*.

There's an old saying that addicts will not get better until they have "hit bottom." This is in many ways an unfortunate adage because it conjures up highly negative images and makes it sound as though addicts can't get better until they have lost their families and jobs and have become homeless and destitute. In fact, addicts will get better as soon as they perceive that the costs of using outweigh the benefits. You could perhaps call any such moment "hitting bottom," but it's probably not a very helpful way to describe it.

TWO STRATEGIES

There are two principal formalized strategies that family members can use to persuade an addict that the costs outweigh the benefits.

One strategy consists of family members having a meeting and expressing love for the addict, but also confronting him or her and communicating hard truths and serious threats as to what will happen if the addictive behavior continues. The idea is that the experience will crash down all at once like a hammer on the costs side of the scale. When this strategy is used in a formal way, it's called an intervention.

The other strategy is much subtler and is designed to change the way the addict views the costs and benefits. Family members adjust their behavior so as to increase the benefits to the addict of not using and also take away any impediments to the person's experiencing the full costs of the addiction. This strategy has been formalized into something called Community Reinforcement and Family Training, or CRAFT.

This chapter will explain the two techniques. As a general comment, interventions can sometimes produce quick positive outcomes, but they tend to work well only in certain specific family situations. CRAFT techniques can take much longer to show results, but they can be used in almost any situation and can be used effectively by one family member even if others are not fully on board.

As another general comment, it often takes family members a very long time to come to these techniques. At the beginning, it seems impossible to believe that a family member can't simply "fix" the problem through the normal persuasive approaches of reasoning, pleading, bargaining, shaming, and so on. After all, the harm is obvious, and the solution seems easy and obvious as well. It often takes many months or years of trying these more traditional approaches before a family member finally gives up and comes to the realization, through long experience, that they don't work.

But this is not wasted time. It's part of the process. Very few people are able to throw themselves wholeheartedly into a counterintuitive technique such as CRAFT unless they have seen *through their own eyes* that more obvious approaches do not produce results.

Finally, it's good to be aware that interventions and CRAFT rely on different assumptions and that professionals who are trained in one technique are sometimes very biased against the other one. In particular, advocates for CRAFT often take the view that interventions can actually be harmful and counterproductive.

WHAT'S AN INTERVENTION?

An intervention is a meeting in which an addict is confronted by a group that may include family members, friends, coworkers, and even religious and community leaders. In recent years, the idea was popularized by a television show called *Intervention*, in which each episode documented such a meeting.

Typically, at the meeting the group does three things:

1. Each member tells the addict that he or she has a problem and describes specific negative behaviors of the addict and how they have affected the member and made the member feel.
2. The group offers a specific treatment plan to the addict, usually involving inpatient detox and rehab, which is to begin immediately.
3. The members describe the specific actions they will take if the addict doesn't accept the treatment offer (i.e., they make threats).

The meeting is usually set up so that it comes as a complete surprise to the addict, making it harder for him or her to simply avoid it. (For this reason, interventions are sometimes ironically referred to as "surprise parties.")

The goal is to break through addicts' denial and put so much weight on the costs side of the scale that they break down and agree to accept treatment. Assuming they say yes, a plan is in place to transport them immediately to a treatment facility, so they don't have a chance to change their mind.

An intervention is often coordinated by an addiction counselor. Some counselors are specially trained for this purpose and are called "interventionists." In addition to preparing the members of the group and arranging the treatment plan, the interventionist may be present to "preside" at the meeting.

While the meeting comes as a surprise to the addict, it usually requires weeks of planning, not only to get a treatment plan in place but also to decide who will attend, find a time and place that works for everyone, figure out how to get the addict there without suspecting an ambush, and educate all the members on how to behave and what to say.

Preparation of the members is key. Ideally, members will express love and support for the addict, but be uncompromising about the fact that the addict has a problem and about the need for treatment. Members should present a united front. If one member becomes angry and accusative (which will make the addict defensive), or if one member starts to waffle about the seriousness of the problem, the chances that the addict will agree to treatment are greatly reduced.

A great deal of thought also needs to be put into the threats. Threats should not be vague (such as "I won't love you anymore"). They should be highly specific, actionable, and serious enough to get the addict's attention. Threats might include no longer allowing the addict to live in the home, withdrawing financial support, divorce or separation, the loss of a job, starting legal proceedings to take away the addict's children, or starting involuntary civil commitment proceedings.

Of course, lesser threats might work, too. The key is that, whatever threats the members come up with, they have to be willing to go through with them. There's always a chance that addicts will call the members' bluff and refuse to go into treatment, or go but then quickly drop out or relapse. If this happens and the members don't carry out their threats, this teaches addicts that they don't really need to worry and that their actions don't have real-world consequences—which will only end up reinforcing their addictive tendencies.

There is no standard length for a meeting. In practice, many last from an hour to an hour and a half, although some can last four to six hours or more if the addict is truly torn about what to do.

DO INTERVENTIONS WORK?

There's no solid statistical evidence yet concerning how often interventions work. When they're done correctly, they can have a high rate of success in getting an addict to agree to go into treatment. The problem is that they sometimes have a lower rate of success in actually getting the addict well.

When addicts find themselves in rehab as the result of an intervention, they're often not particularly motivated to use the program and in fact might be full of resentment about being there in the first place. After all, they didn't freely choose to be there. (If you think of addiction as putting an unfair thumb on the benefits side of the scale, an intervention is a bit like putting an unfair thumb on the costs side of the scale. The two might balance each other out, but the addict is still not making a free and independent choice.)

That's not to say that rehab can't work. In fact, statistics show that addiction treatments can be quite successful even if the addict hasn't freely chosen to participate. The intervention experience, the rehab environment, and the simple fact of being separated from their substance of choice are often enough to persuade addicts after a while that they do have a problem and should try to get better. However, there's no question that rehab is more likely to succeed if the addict is highly motivated to make it work upon arrival.

Perhaps the biggest problem with interventions is that they tend to work only if the members of the group are on the same page or if the interventionist can succeed in getting them on the same page. Sometimes key family members are so angry or hurt that they can't approach the meeting with the calmness and rationality it requires and end up turning it into an unproductive fight. Sometimes key family members are themselves in denial about the problem or engaging in enabling behavior, which can give the addict an "out."

And of course, sometimes the members can't agree on the threats or can't be trusted to actually carry them out if necessary. In fact, a significant number of families who begin planning an intervention decide not to go through with it simply because they find the prospect of having to carry out a truly effective threat (such as turning the addict out of the home) too difficult to bear.

There are enough stories of failed interventions in popular culture that some people believe that interventions rarely work. But a better way of thinking about them is by analogy to medicine, where there are treatments that tend to be successful only for certain types of patients or in certain situations. Patients who meet all the criteria are said to be "good candidates" for the treatment because there is a good chance that the treatment will work *for them*. In the same way, interventions are not for everyone. They can work well, but they tend to be successful only if the addict and the family meet the criteria and qualify as "good candidates."

It should also be noted that a failed intervention—where the addict refuses to get help—can leave the addict with a deep sense of betrayal and sometimes exacerbate the problem. In addition, even when an intervention is *successful* and the addict ends up in long-term recovery, it's not uncommon for the addict to feel bitterness and resentment for a long time over the fact of the intervention and the way it was carried out. The experience of an intervention can be deeply painful, and the mere fact of being in recovery doesn't necessarily erase the pain.

HOW TO FIND AN INTERVENTIONIST

It's not absolutely necessary to have an interventionist preside at the meeting, but a professional can often help keep things on track when the addict tries to derail the process through distractions and deflections. A professional is also a very good idea if the addict has any history of other mental illnesses or of violent or suicidal tendencies.

You may be able to get a referral to an interventionist through a local mental health treatment facility. There is also a professional organization called the Association of Intervention Specialists, or AIS. You can find a list of its members, organized by state, at its website, *www. associationofinterventionspecialists.org.*

AIS members who have completed a training program, have at least two years of experience, and meet certain other criteria can receive the BRI-I certification. There is also a BRI-II certification, which requires a minimum of five years of experience and additional training in behavioral addictions such as gambling, sex, and shopping.

It's a good idea to ask about an interventionist's qualifications and experience. Professionals who are not members of AIS might still be well qualified if they have experience and a relevant degree. Many interventionists are psychologists or have a master's degree or doctorate in social work (MSW, DSW, or PhD). A licensed clinical social worker (LCSW) is someone with at least an MSW who specializes in mental health issues.

TIPS FOR A SUCCESSFUL INTERVENTION

Some suggestions for a successful intervention include:

- Allow sufficient time to prepare all the members. If an addict is engaged in truly self-destructive behavior, you might need to take other steps to keep him or her safe in the meantime, but don't rush the intervention and leave the group members unprepared.
- Invite only people whom the addict genuinely likes and respects. For instance, coworkers might have a great perspective on the effects of the addict's actions, but if the addict doesn't think highly of them, he or she is more likely to resist.
- If a key member ought to be included, but you're afraid the person will sabotage the intervention by becoming angry or waffling, one idea is to have the person write a short statement that can be read at the meeting by someone else.
- Stage a rehearsal. This allows you to decide who will speak in what order, where everyone will sit, and so on, so there's no fumbling or confusion when the time comes.
- A rehearsal is a great time to anticipate the addict's objections and arguments and formulate responses to them. You can also

discuss preparing emotionally for an addict's anger and accusations of betrayal.

- When choosing a time for the meeting, the emphasis should be on finding a time when the addict is least likely to be drunk or high. It's also good to choose a place where the addict will feel at home and comfortable.
- When speaking, you can limit an addict's arguing back by sticking to describing specific incidents and how they made you feel, as opposed to making generalized statements about the addict that he or she can deny. It's also helpful to write your statement out in advance.
- Demand an immediate decision. The intervention is the time when you have maximum leverage. Don't give the addict a few days to think it over or you're less likely to get a yes.
- To avoid giving addicts time to change their mind about going to treatment, it can be a good idea to have already packed a suitcase. Packing can take a long time and make the process seem more "real" to the addict.

OTHER INTERVENTION ISSUES

One-Person Interventions

Sometimes single individuals on whom an addict is highly dependent can stage what is in effect an intervention all by themselves. For instance, a spouse or parent may tell an addict that he or she must go to treatment immediately or be thrown out of the house. This can work, if the ultimatum is serious enough and if the addict believes that the person is willing to go through with the threat.

However, if it's possible, involving other like-minded people can greatly increase the pressure on the addict and put a lot less pressure on the person staging the intervention.

Multiple Interventions

Sometimes an intervention is initially successful—the addict goes to treatment and is better for a time—but after a while he or she relapses and refuses to get further help. Should the family attempt a second intervention?

Multiple interventions have been known to work, but in general their success rate is low. After all, there's no reason to think that the second intervention will work better than the first one, especially since the "shock value" of the experience will be greatly lessened because the addict has been through it before.

A better approach is usually to simply carry out the threats made at the first intervention. If the threats were well crafted to begin with, they should be enough to get the addict's attention.

Alternative Interventions

The traditional intervention described in this chapter is sometimes referred to as a Johnson Institute intervention. The model was pioneered by Dr. Vernon Johnson in the 1960s.

Since then, there have been a few alternative approaches that are designed to lessen the severity and possible feelings of shock and betrayal associated with the traditional model. For instance, the Albany-Rochester Interventional Sequence for Engagement, or ARISE, intervention differs from the standard model in that there is no "surprise." The addict is told that the family will meet and that he or she can attend or not. The hope is to elicit the addict's cooperation without a dramatic confrontation. If the addict refuses, the family can engage in further strategies up to and including a traditional Johnson-style intervention.

Another technique is the systemic family model intervention. The focus here is on the way addiction affects a family. The entire family is invited to a series of meetings with a professional, at which they discuss how addiction affects family members and how family members' reactions affect the addict in turn. The addict is encouraged to get treatment, but the family members are also encouraged to seek out therapy or support groups.

WHAT IS CRAFT?

The main difference between the intervention approach and the CRAFT approach is that interventions rely on a dramatic confrontation, whereas CRAFT believes that confrontations and threats are almost always counterproductive. According to CRAFT, reacting to an addict with confrontation (or yelling, sulking, or other negative behavior) not only doesn't tend to work but actually reinforces addictive behavior by making addicts feel angry, hurt, and resentful and giving them an excuse to use substances. And while an intervention might force an addict into some form of treatment, CRAFT believes that it is less likely to result in a positive outcome over the long term.

CRAFT derives from a psychological theory called behaviorism, which was pioneered by Harvard psychologist B. F. Skinner. In contrast to traditional Freudian psychoanalysis, which sought to explain certain behaviors by means of obscure processes in the unconscious, Skinner believed that behavior could be understood much more simply as a reaction to rewards and punishments in the environment. Change the rewards and punishments, he thought, and you change behavior. Simple as that. (Well, not quite as simple as that, but that was the basic principle.)

The main idea of CRAFT is that if you want addicts to change their behavior, you don't just tell them what you want them to do; you start by changing *your* behavior so as to adjust the rewards and punishments in the environment. In effect, you change the outcome of the cost-benefit scale by (1) adding new benefits for not using and (2) eliminating confrontation and creating different and more effective costs for using.

Back in the 1970s a group of behaviorists developed a method of helping addicts in recovery called the Community Reinforcement Approach. Rather than focusing on the addicts' inner psychological workings, this approach sought to adjust their environment and give them practical skills to cope with life without alcohol or drugs. Examples included helping addicts find jobs, get marriage counseling, plan their leisure time, find sober friends, and so on.

Robert Meyers, a member of the group, expanded the idea to help families of addicts who weren't in recovery and were refusing to accept treatment, ultimately developing the CRAFT strategy.

CRAFT is complicated, but at its core it teaches families to influence an addict's behavior in three ways: positive communication, positive reinforcement, and allowing natural consequences.

Positive Communication

CRAFT believes that negative communication—criticizing, confronting, expressing frustration, and so on—doesn't help and in fact makes the problem worse. Thus it encourages family members to communicate with an addict only in a positive way.

Among other things, this means praising addicts for what they do right rather than criticizing them for what they do wrong, and telling them what you want them to do (such as chores around the house) rather than nagging them about what you don't want them to do.

Positive communication means not letting an addict bait you into a fight. General guidelines for communication include being brief, being highly specific, and using "I" statements (such as "I feel afraid when . . ." as opposed to "You are so inconsiderate . . ."). When possible, it means expressing some understanding of what the addict is experiencing, accepting partial responsibility for situations, and offering to help or work together.

The general idea is not to express anger at the addict and not to communicate in such a way that the addict can get mad at you. When addicts can no longer use the family as a verbal punching bag or use family frustrations as an excuse to drink or use, they are forced to confront more directly the reality of their situation.

Needless to say, this is highly difficult to pull off. Family members often feel tremendous anger, frustration, and fear, and they want most of all for the addict to acknowledge their feelings. But CRAFT teaches them to behave with a certain falseness, setting aside those feelings and acting according to a different script.

In fact, the analogy to acting is no exaggeration. People trained in CRAFT often work with families to role-play situations so they can practice their comments and reactions. Family members are urged to write down what they plan to say to an addict and practice it in advance. The promised payoff is that different behavior on the family's part will result in different behavior on the addict's part.

Positive Reinforcement

CRAFT teaches family members to come up with positive reinforcements for good behavior on the addict's part. If the addict doesn't drink on a particular occasion or does something otherwise thoughtful and positive, he or she can be rewarded. It's not necessary to make the reward system explicit; rather, addicts can simply discover on their own that good things follow good behavior.

Rewards don't have to be elaborate or expensive. They can be as simple as a nice comment or a moment of affection. They could also include things the addict likes—going to a movie or a favorite dinner, for instance.

While CRAFT believes in rewards, it doesn't believe in punishment—an addict should never be punished for bad behavior, only rewarded for good behavior. However, if an addict engages in bad behavior, the family can withdraw the reward—as long as it does so in a matter-of-fact way, not a punitive way. ("Since you're drinking tonight, I'd rather not go to the movie, but I hope we can see it another time.")

If this sounds a lot like training a dog to do tricks, well . . . honestly, it is. It's the same basic technique used by professional animal trainers. Trainers reward good behavior and simply ignore bad behavior. They reward small steps in the right direction and give bigger rewards for bigger steps. CRAFT just takes the same idea and applies it to dealing with addiction.

Natural Consequences

While CRAFT doesn't believe in punishment, it does believe in getting out of the way and allowing addicts to experience the natural consequences of their actions, rather than covering for them, making excuses for them, or trying to make everything "all right."

As people slide into addiction, they tend to engage in actions (or failures to act) that result in a lot of unfortunate consequences. They may be late for appointments, sleep through activities, overspend, pass out on the floor, alienate friends, or forget important responsibilities. It's very natural for families to respond by trying to take care of the person—making excuses, taking on their missed responsibilities, or dragging them into bed.

CRAFT suggests that it's often better *not* to take care of such people—in other words, not to engage in enabling—and instead to let them experience the natural consequences of what they do. After all, if addicts find that no matter how irresponsible they are, their family will make everything work out, they are being trained to believe that it's okay to be irresponsible. By letting them sleep through things they want to do, wake up on the living room floor, or face the consequences of forgetting their responsibilities, addicts will instead have to confront the reality of their condition. The natural consequences themselves start to put a weight on the costs side of the scale.

Natural consequences don't count as "punishment" because you're not imposing them on the addict. You're simply stepping out of the way and letting them happen. It's much harder for addicts to get mad at you, since you literally didn't do anything to hurt them.

The problem with allowing natural consequences is that it can be hard to draw the line. You don't want to allow consequences that could truly be unsafe (such as allowing someone to drive drunk). And you don't want to allow consequences that are as difficult for you as they are for the addict (such as allowing one spouse to gamble away money that both spouses need). It can take a lot of thought to decide which consequences you can live with allowing.

DOES CRAFT WORK?

The basic idea of CRAFT is to change the way the addict perceives the cost-benefit scale. Certainly, allowing natural consequences adds weight to the "costs" side of the scale. But you've also introduced a new wrinkle—through positive communication and reinforcement, you've created benefits for *not* using, whereas the addict before only thought in terms of the benefits of using.

Does CRAFT succeed in getting addicts into treatment? In many cases, it does. It's not nearly as quick as an intervention, and it requires making major, difficult changes in your life, while acting in ways that might strike some people as false or manipulative. On the plus side, CRAFT is designed not to threaten addicts into treatment they don't want, but to gradually persuade them to decide for themselves to go into treatment they *do* want. As a result, the treatment prognosis might be more positive.

As a side benefit, a great many people who practice CRAFT techniques find that, once they get used to them, they make their home life much more manageable while they are waiting for an addict to get help. (Indeed, the mere fact of having a strategy to guide one's behavior, as opposed to simply careening from one crisis to another, can in and of itself relieve a great deal of stress.)

There have been a handful of scientific studies regarding the effectiveness of CRAFT. Most of these have been rather small, ranging from a dozen to about a hundred people. Overall, the studies suggest that CRAFT is very effective at getting addicts into treatment and is also successful at improving the reported quality of life of family members who practice it. A few comparative studies suggest that CRAFT has a better statistical success rate than interventions.

There are a few downsides to CRAFT, however. One is that it can take a long time—many months or even years. In cases where addicts are truly a danger to themselves or others, families might not have the luxury of this kind of time. That's also true where the addict is the family's sole breadwinner and is in danger of losing his or her job.

Another downside is that CRAFT sometimes backfires with opioid addicts. Unlike many alcoholics, opioid addicts can be much more pleasant and cooperative when they're high and exhibit nasty behaviors only when they enter withdrawal. As a result, families that use positive reinforcement for "good" behavior can end up unwittingly rewarding the very actions they are trying to prevent. (Also, allowing natural consequences by refusing to intervene when an addict passes out can be very dangerous with an opioid user, who could suffer an overdose.)

Finally, a common complaint about CRAFT is that it appears to amount to rewarding people for behaving badly and requires treating family members who cause problems more nicely than family members who don't. As one spouse said, "If this works, I'll end up married to a sober narcissist."

But another way of looking at it is that CRAFT isn't about rewarding addiction; it's about finding a way of communicating effectively with someone whose normal reasoning and decision-making skills have been impaired. Most of us naturally adjust our communication styles when we're around small children or older people with dementia; we know that we can't successfully interact with them as we would with a healthy adult. In the same way, it can be helpful for families to change the way they interact with an addict. The reason it seems unnatural to do so is that it's so easy to forget that the addict is psychologically impaired. That's because an addict (unlike someone with Alzheimer's disease) is impaired in only one specific aspect of life—and is usually doing everything that he or she can precisely to cover up that fact.

More information about interventions and CRAFT can be found in the Resources at the back of the book.

· · · · · · · 13 · · · · · · ·

How to Cope When a Loved One Is Refusing Treatment

Addiction is a problem that affects the whole family, but it often seems as though only one member of the family is getting any attention—the addict.

Living with a person in active addiction—who is in denial or otherwise refusing to go to treatment—can be a nightmare. It's as though the addict sucks up all the oxygen in the house and everyone else's lives and routines are left in pieces. Family members often become obsessed with the addict and stop paying attention to their own needs. They become casualties of the addiction, collateral damage in its wake.

Needless to say, this is unhealthy behavior. One of the most important things that family members need to learn to do—and also one of the hardest—is to continue taking care of themselves. Among other things, this includes getting enough sleep and exercise, eating well, seeing friends, and scheduling time for recreation and relaxation.

Many family members will say, "That's impossible! I'm too worried." Others will say they feel too guilty to schedule dinner and a movie with friends while a loved one is at home drinking or off using drugs.

But the truth is, if family members are at their wits' end, they're not in good shape to help an addict. Family members who are able to stay healthy and relatively well adjusted among the tumult will be much more capable of eventually guiding addicts into treatment and taking care of them in the meantime. It's far better if only one member of a family is sick and debilitated than if every member of the family is.

You've probably heard the familiar airplane safety instructions at the start of each flight. During the part about oxygen masks, after explaining how to use and adjust the masks, the instructions always say, "Be sure to put on your own mask before helping others."

Why? Because if you're getting enough oxygen yourself, you're better able to help a child or an elderly person. If you try to help the other person first—especially if the other person is confused or upset—you might pass out before you succeed. There's a risk that you both will run out of air. It's the same problem with addiction: If you're not taking care of yourself first, you're less able to care for the addict. Looking out for your own safety first is *not* selfishness; it's actually the best way to care for someone else.

To take another example, did you know that a very large part of life-guards' training is not about how to rescue a drowning person, but about how lifeguards can avoid being drowned themselves during a rescue? That's because people who get into trouble in the water and start to panic will instinctively grab onto anything nearby—including a lifeguard—and push it down into the water in an effort to pull themselves up. Lifeguards spend a lot of time training in how not to drown in this way.

People who attempt to rescue a drowning person without such training are at great risk of dying themselves—so much so, in fact, that there's a name for the phenomenon: AVIR syndrome, for "aquatic victim instead of rescuer."

In the same way, addicts who are actively suffering from the disease will often blame or hurt those close to them in a panicky effort to cope with their problems. A lot of family members who try to "rescue" an addict are also in danger of getting hurt themselves instead of providing assistance. It's fine to try to help, of course, but it's critical to look after yourself and make sure that you don't get hurt in the process—that you don't experience "addiction victim instead of rescuer" syndrome.

WHAT YOU CAN DO

Taking care of yourself in the tension-filled environment of addiction is clearly easier said than done. No one does it perfectly; it's impossible to imagine someone living around an addict in a peaceful oasis of calm. But making *some* effort is better than nothing. Anything you can do to set aside time for yourself is helpful. And that often begins with making a decision not to feel guilty about doing so and to understand that in the long run it is helpful not only to you but to the addict as well.

Finding a therapist, social worker, or other professional who is familiar with addiction to talk to can be a good step. While you might be tempted to try to bring the addict into the therapy, it's good to remember that you need someone to talk to *yourself* about your own experiences and feelings. Addiction is a family disease, and you need your own form of recovery. The goal is to heal yourself in the process of trying to heal someone else.

It can also be helpful to join a support group, so that you can share stories with people who are undergoing similar experiences. Many people find that this gives them a great deal of strength and guidance in dealing with a family crisis.

Al-Anon is the most well-known such group, but there are others, and they have different philosophies and approaches. If possible, it can be good to try a number of groups to see where you feel most comfortable. Contact information for these groups can be found in the Resources at the back of the book.

AL-ANON
· ·

Al-Anon was founded in 1951 and is basically Alcoholics Anonymous for family members. In fact, one of the founders of Al-Anon was the wife of a founder of AA.

A key premise of Al-Anon is that alcoholism is a family problem and the family members of an alcoholic need help recovering in the same way that alcoholics need help recovering. For this reason, Al-Anon members are supposed to practice the Twelve Steps, applying them to their own situation. For example, family members are supposed to begin by admitting that they are powerless over alcohol, acknowledging that their lives are unmanageable, and giving themselves over to a higher power.

The actual practice and format of Al-Anon meetings is extremely similar to that of AA meetings. (See Chapter 29 for a detailed description of AA meetings.)

The focus of Al-Anon is on helping the family member—*not* on helping the alcoholic or getting the alcoholic into treatment. There is a common saying in Al-Anon that "changed attitudes aid recovery," but the primary emphasis is on helping the family regardless of whether the alcoholic ever achieves recovery.

In fact, a fundamental philosophical principle of Al-Anon is that a family member *cannot* in the end exert much of an influence over an alcoholic's behavior. A common Al-Anon saying is "I didn't cause it, I can't control it, and I can't cure it." Al-Anon tends to believe that a big part of the family disease of addiction is the family members' mistaken belief that they are somehow responsible for the alcoholic's drinking and are able to make it stop. This mistaken belief is what leads to frustration, guilt, anger, and hopelessness. By giving up the idea that the family is responsible for the problem and able to affect it, family members can be restored to some measure of sanity. (And, paradoxically, this sanity might even help the alcoholic as well.)

Al-Anon is an overwhelmingly female organization. A 2006 survey conducted by Al-Anon of its members in the United States and Canada showed that 85 percent were women. Some observers have suggested that the group's themes of overcoming low self-esteem and self-blame tend to resonate particularly with a female demographic.

OTHER TWELVE-STEP GROUPS

Closely related to Al-Anon is Alateen, a group founded by Al-Anon for family members who are teenagers. The group's 2006 survey showed that 65 percent of Alateen members are female.

Some other groups have sprung up that use the basic Al-Anon model. These include Nar-Anon (for family members of drug addicts), Narateen (the drug equivalent of Alateen), Gam-Anon (for family members of gambling addicts), and Co-Dependents Anonymous.

Families Anonymous is another large Twelve-Step organization, although it is not affiliated with Al-Anon or Nar-Anon. The group was founded in 1971 and offers more than 500 meetings each week in the United States and 12 other countries, including the United Kingdom, Australia, and Canada. It focuses on avoiding codependency, denial, enabling, and similar behaviors.

Adult Children of Alcoholics is a Twelve-Step group that, despite its name, welcomes adult children of drug addicts as well. (See Chapter 16 for more information on this group.)

SMART RECOVERY FAMILY & FRIENDS

SMART Recovery is a support group for addicts that relies on cognitive and behavioral principles and sees itself as an alternative to Alcoholics

Anonymous. (See Chapter 31 for more details.) The organization also offers support groups for addicts' loved ones, called SMART Recovery Family & Friends.

The Family & Friends meetings emphasize the use of CRAFT techniques, especially positive communication, positive reinforcement, and allowing natural consequences. (CRAFT techniques are discussed in more detail in Chapter 12.)

Family & Friends differs from Al-Anon in a number of important ways:

- Family & Friends doesn't use the Twelve Steps and sees itself as based on science rather than spirituality or a belief in a higher power.
- Family & Friends places a greater emphasis on getting the addict into recovery, as opposed to focusing solely on helping the family member feel better emotionally.
- Family & Friends doesn't accept the Al-Anon view that a family member can't control the disease. It attempts to give family members practical tools to reduce addictive behavior.
- Family & Friends meetings include back-and-forth discussions and group problem solving, as opposed to Al-Anon meetings, where members typically speak only once and are discouraged from responding to one another.

EDUCATIONAL GROUPS

A number of groups are designed to provide family members with education about the disease as well as support. There are no truly national organizations that fit this model, but individual groups may be offered by a local facility for treating addiction or mental illness. Calling around to such facilities may provide helpful information.

In the United States, some educational and support groups exist at the state level. For instance, Parents of Addicted Loved Ones operates a number of meetings in Arizona, Indiana, and Kentucky, as well as at least one meeting in about 12 other states. A group called Learn to Cope, which focuses primarily on opioid addiction, has numerous meetings throughout Massachusetts.

14

Dealing with a Child
Who Is an Addict

U nless you have lived through it, there is no way to fully understand the fear, heartsickness, and grief of parents whose child has a terrible affliction. And addiction is one of the most terrible because it doesn't just threaten the child's health; it also alters the child's personality and behavior. The beautiful young person the parents loved and cared for seems no longer to be there and to have been replaced by someone they don't recognize and who can be manipulative and sometimes even cruel.

Every family member of an addict suffers, but people whose addicted loved one is a child tend to suffer certain things more than others. One of these is feelings of guilt. Most parents of addicts frequently wonder to themselves, consciously or unconsciously, "What did I do wrong?" They ransack their memories trying to figure out what they might have done differently to prevent their child from getting sick.

In the vast majority of cases, the answer is "nothing." Short of abusing a child, there's simply nothing most parents can do to increase (or decrease) the chances of a child becoming an addict. There's no hard evidence to suggest that parenting styles affect addiction. Many addicts report very happy childhoods, and a tremendous number of people in recovery will tell you that nothing their parents did or didn't do would have made any difference at all in how their brains reacted to an addictive substance.

But that seldom stops parents from harboring guilt feelings. These can be exacerbated by the fact that children in active addiction tend to become defensive and often lash out and blame parents rather than accept responsibility for their own problems. Furthermore, many friends and relatives who don't fully understand addiction may look on the parents of an addict with suspicion, wondering if they were bad parents or somehow did something to cause the disease.

Another feeling that parents often have is helplessness. When a child is young, parents are the ones who are in charge; they're usually able to step in and fix things and make everything better. When a child develops an addiction, and the parents do absolutely everything they can think of but still can't solve the problem, they often despair and feel inadequate. Furthermore, most parents are used to having their children listen to them and treat them with a measure of respect. When children completely ignore their parents' seemingly sensible advice to stop ruining their life, the parents can feel completely powerless.

Of course, parents are also liable to feel the same things that all family members of addicts tend to feel: stress, anger, obsession, and so on. And like all family members, parents often engage in enabling behaviors, at least at first. In fact, enabling is frequently much more of an issue for parents than for other family members, simply because parents have such a natural instinct to protect their children from harm.

Addiction can be a particularly acute problem if parents don't agree on how to handle the situation. It's very important for parents to present a united front in dealing with the child and to support each other in handling the stress. If one parent is in denial or engaged in enabling and the other one isn't, it can cause tremendous conflicts. Sadly, these conflicts can be made worse by the child's own behavior. Addicted children often become experts at playing one parent off the other and manipulating any disagreements to get their way and be able to continue using.

When parents are divorced or separated, it's even more difficult because they likely don't have the regular communication necessary to present a united front in response to the child. And their own simmering resentments and conflicts may hamper their ability to work together.

It's not unheard of for one parent to simply throw up his or her hands and refuse to deal with the problem at all, dumping everything in the other parent's lap. Some couples even break up over the stress of a child's addiction. (On the other hand, some couples are brought closer together by the need to deal with the crisis.)

When discussing how to deal with addicted children, the first question is usually whether or not the child is living at home, because this makes an enormous difference.

CHILDREN LIVING AT HOME

Research shows that the most common age for the onset of alcoholism is 18 to 19. It's certainly possible to develop the problem earlier or later, although statistically the likelihood decreases significantly after age 25. As for opioids, one study found that the average age of first use is between 25 and 26. So, commonly, when parents first start dealing with an addicted child, that child is a teenager or a young adult. (Of course, children can develop an addiction in their 30s or 40s, especially if they do so as a result of exposure to prescription painkillers, and some children who develop an addiction early are still struggling with it many years later, so parents often have to deal with the problem well into adulthood.)

Many addicted children are living at home, either because they never left the nest or because their ability to keep up the responsibilities of living independently fell apart after the addiction kicked in.

There aren't a lot of statistics on how many addicted children live with their parents. (In the United States, compiling meaningful statistics is difficult because there has been a recent sharp increase in the number of adults living with their parents for other reasons, such as difficulty finding a job or high student loan debt.) However, while you might think that addicted children would want to live anywhere other than under parental supervision, the truth is that a significant number of such children *want* to live with their parents. In many ways it's an ideal situation for maintaining an addiction: Living at home often allows them to avoid the responsibilities of cooking, housework, and paying rent. Parents are often understanding and easy to manipulate. And since most parents work during the day, sleep at night, and have other responsibilities, addicts are frequently able to escape direct supervision for all but a few hours a week.

Of course, there are also many addicted children who don't want to live with their parents but have no other practical choice.

Either way, having an addicted child living at home can cause enormous conflicts for a family. If the child doesn't have a full-time job—which is likely the case—he or she may keep very different hours from the parents and may behave very disruptively. The addiction may cause defensiveness, fight-picking, and nastiness. Addicted children tend to behave immaturely in general because the problem interferes with the development of the prefrontal cortex, which largely governs mature decision making.

An addicted child may bring undesirable friends into the house, especially when the parents are out, leading the parents to feel that they're no longer in charge of their own home. And the parents may be very worried about the presence of illegal drugs in the house—particularly if they have jobs such as a nurse or a law enforcement officer, where the discovery of drugs in their home could have negative employment consequences.

The situation is even worse if parents have other children living at home. The other children's lives may be severely disrupted as well, including their schoolwork, sleep, social life, and mental well-being. Parents may be very upset about having illegal drugs in the house around their other children. And the presence of the addicted child often leads to fights and tension between the other children or between the other children and the addict or the parents.

Many parents try to deal with these problems by setting rules for the addicted child—no drugs on the premises, no guests without permission, a curfew, and so on. Parents might also require the child to pay rent, as a way of forcing him or her to straighten up and get a job. Some parents have even drawn up a written contract and asked their child to sign it.

The problem, of course, is that addicted children will typically agree to all the parents' conditions—and then completely ignore them. Even if the children meant well at the time, their prefrontal cortex has been impaired, and so their ability to rationally "live by the rules" regarding substances has been hijacked and dismantled.

If parents repeatedly let children get away with breaking the rules, the children will learn that the rules are meaningless and that breaking them has no consequences. As a result, the children will have no incentive to get well because they can continue to abuse substances and still have all their needs taken care of for them.

Rules make sense only if the parents are prepared to enforce them. And sadly, in most cases, the only way to enforce the rules is with a credible threat that if they're not adhered to, the child will lose the privilege of living at home.

THREATENING TO KICK A CHILD OUT

Parents naturally recoil at the idea of kicking a child out of the house. They fear that the child will become homeless, get sick, and perhaps die. The weight of their guilt is impossible to convey.

Nevertheless, it's reasonable for parents to set rules to preserve their own sanity and quality of life. Addicts have no right to destroy their parents' lives. And parents with more than one child have to consider the other children, too—parents have a duty to take care of *all* their children, not just the addicted one.

Sooner or later, many parents end up contemplating the "natural consequence" of not allowing a child to live at home unless he or she agrees to go into treatment. (This is a bit like an intervention, except that it involves only the parents and only one specific threat.)

Faced with the prospect of not being able to live at home, many children will agree to treatment. Some children will refuse and move out. In many cases, the child will embark on a period of couch-surfing and rough living and will eventually return home and agree to treatment once he or she has exhausted the good will of friends and acquaintances.

Many parents report that not allowing a child to live at home was the critical first step in getting the child well.

However, there's no question that it's dangerous and uncertain for addicted children to live on their own. Whether to take this step—whether allowing children to live at home is enabling them or just sensibly protecting them—is an incredibly heart-wrenching decision for a parent to make.

But here's a thought: All children at some point need to "launch." The job of parents is, in a sense, to raise their children so that someday they no longer need parenting. This is difficult for *all* parents, not just parents of addicts. All parents have difficulty letting go; all parents worry that their children will have difficulty making it on their own and have many difficult life lessons ahead of them. Parents of addicts simply face a much more extreme example of a universal phenomenon. Such parents may believe that their children are not yet capable of acting responsibly—*and they may be completely right*—but on the other hand, there's only one way to learn to take responsibility for your actions, and that's to start being forced to do so.

BOYFRIENDS AND GIRLFRIENDS

It's not uncommon for addicted children to have boyfriends or girl-friends who are also addicts, or at least heavy substance abusers. If the child is living at home, these boyfriends or girlfriends may spend a lot of time at the parents' house—particularly if they don't have a good domestic situation themselves.

While parents generally try to be accepting of their children's romantic choices, it's hard to avoid the conclusion that a romance between two addicts is unlikely to be a healthy, mutually beneficial relationship. It's more likely to be one that reinforces each other's bad habits. At best, parents may feel that the boyfriend or girlfriend is a potential bad influence on the child. At worst, they may feel that the significant other is a destructive force, one that is preying on the child, supplying the child with drugs, or keeping him or her from getting help.

Parents often resent the presence of the boyfriend or girlfriend in their house, especially if they have other children at home who may be upset or negatively affected by the person.

One of the "rules" that some parents adopt is that the boyfriend or girlfriend isn't allowed in the house. The question is what the conse-quences should be for breaking this rule. If parents aren't willing to bar their own child from their house for breaking this rule, then there are some alternatives.

Some parents have obtained restraining orders against a child's boyfriend or girlfriend. This effectively bars the person from the house by legal means. The problem is that many jurisdictions allow restraining orders to be filed only by relatives or roommates of the restrained person or require proof of actual or threatened physical harm. This makes them unavailable in most cases.

Another option is to obtain a no-trespassing order. In the United States, the procedure varies by state, but it generally involves informing the police about the person, posting signs on your property, and issuing a warning to the person or having the police issue the warning. If the boyfriend or girlfriend shows up despite the warning, the parents can call the police and have the person arrested.

CHILDREN NOT LIVING AT HOME

Addicted children who are not living at home pose a different set of problems.

In some cases a child has an addiction but is managing to hold down a job and an apartment or is managing to get by living with friends. In other cases a child has "launched" successfully and may have a spouse and a family and has only recently developed an addiction. And some older children who are living independently are being supported by their parents as they struggle to work through their problems.

For parents in this situation, the main problem is usually a lack of information. Because they don't see their children every day, they may have little idea of how they're doing and what they need. The uncertainty often becomes a gnawing worry.

If the child has a spouse or significant other who is not an addict, then it may be helpful to try to enlist that person as a kind of "third parent." Parents and spouses presenting a united front can be very helpful, and open communication between them can help to resolve issues. Unfortunately, it's not uncommon for addicted children to manipulate a spouse or significant other to prevent this from happening. If the parents are intent on getting a child into treatment, the child may persuade the spouse that the parents are interfering or meddling and shouldn't be listened to.

Children who aren't living at home but are suffering from an addiction often end up approaching their parents for some form of support, particularly financial support. The addiction may prevent them from successfully holding down a job, or they may need money to support their habit. This can pose a dilemma for parents because it's not always clear when providing support amounts to enabling.

Refusing to provide financial support, or conditioning it on the addict's getting treatment, may be useful in getting the addict to accept help. However, it can be hard for a parent to say "no," particularly when a child makes a frantic call asking for money for food or to forestall eviction. No parent wants to refuse a child in these circumstances, but on the other hand, the parent may have no idea if the child is telling the truth about the situation. And even if the child *does* need money for food or rent, the parent might fear that the child will still use the money for drugs instead.

Some parents agree to help a child but insist on paying bills directly rather than simply giving the child cash.

In the end, this is another hard decision, and only the parents themselves can decide where to draw the line between protecting their children and enabling them.

IF A CHILD AGREES TO TREATMENT

If a child agrees to treatment, the next step is finding an appropriate treatment plan. Some parents work out a treatment plan themselves in advance and present it to the child, perhaps as an alternative to being pushed out of the house or as a condition of receiving financial support. On the other hand, some parents prefer to have their children research and find a treatment plan themselves (as long as it's acceptable to the parents), reasoning that the children need to demonstrate responsibility and will be more likely to succeed at a program that they have picked out on their own.

If the plan involves rehab or a sober-living arrangement, one possibility to consider is a facility in another state, or at least one that's a long distance away. Living close to home can present a newly recovering addict with a great many triggers—people, places, and things that are associated with substance use and that can create a temptation to relapse. Being in a very different environment can sometimes be helpful in allowing the person to start a new life.

If an addicted child is on the young side, it can be helpful to find a program that specializes in teens or young adults. Children may feel more at home and enthusiastic in a program that puts them with their peers, and interactions with people the same age in therapy and support groups can often be helpful.

• • • • • • • 15 • • • • • • •

Dealing with a Spouse
Who Is an Addict

Spouses of addicts generally feel all the same things that other family members feel—anger, stress, guilt, obsession, and so on. But they also feel something else, or at least they feel it in a different way, and that is a deep sense of *betrayal*.

Addiction is in many ways similar to infidelity. The addicted spouse has abandoned the other spouse and taken up with a new love—a substance. The addicted spouse cares about the substance much more than about the other spouse. The addicted spouse is faithful to the substance and dismissive or abusive toward the other spouse. The other spouse ends up feeling as though an interloper has entered the marital relationship and taken over his or her rightful place.

This is not a mere metaphor. The feelings that spouses experience—jealousy, rage, deep emotional hurt—are exactly the same as those experienced when someone is unfaithful.

Of course, addiction is different from infidelity because the addicted spouse isn't acting with intent. It's simply a disease. And the other spouse may know—intellectually—that that's true, but it doesn't make the hurt any less or any differently.

In fact, the hurt of addiction may be even worse than the hurt of infidelity.

Spouses who are unfaithful are generally aware of what they're doing and how it might affect the betrayed spouse. They might be sorry and feel remorse. They might apologize. They might feel guilty and try to treat the other spouse better. They might learn to value their marriage more highly.

Addicts, on the other hand, tend to be in denial about their problems and their effect on others. They can't learn to value their marriage more highly than their substance because their brain is sending them the opposite message. Because they are blocking out what they do wrong, they are less likely to express regret and understanding. What's more, they tend to be highly defensive. They're likely to lash out at the spouse and blame the spouse for causing their problems. They may do this proactively, even if the spouse has done nothing to provoke it.

YOU ALWAYS HURT THE ONE YOU LOVE

Addicts tend to train their vituperative firepower the hardest at the people they're closest to and trust the most. That's because these are the people who they think are least likely to abandon or hurt them despite their misbehavior. And most often, the person who comes in for the heaviest verbal gunfire is a spouse. What's worse, the more loving and caring spouses are, the worse addicts are likely to treat them, simply because they have come to believe that this is the one person they can count on.

When addicts want to deflect blame or change the subject, the surest way to do so is to push the other person's buttons—to turn the subject to issues the other person is most sensitive about. Spouses tend to know each other's buttons much better than anyone else's. For this reason, addicts can inflict psychological pain on a spouse extremely effectively.

The result of all of this is that addiction can often lead to divorce or separation.

In the past, it was traditional for married couples to promise to care for each other "in sickness and in health." Indeed, most people would consider it cruel for someone to abandon a spouse just because he or she developed a physical disease such as cancer. And even with an illness such as Alzheimer's disease, which (like addiction) alters a spouse's personality and diminishes the ability to be fully present in a marriage, there are countless spouses who faithfully care for their loved ones during their decline. Addiction, however, is different. Alzheimer's disease is profoundly sad, but it doesn't tend to send spouses into a jealous rage or make them feel deeply emotionally betrayed.

Obviously, an addict's behavior can become so unbearable that a spouse may simply find it impossible to continue to live with the addict. That's a decision that spouses have to make for themselves; no one else can put themselves in a spouse's position.

For spouses who choose to stay, though, one thing that's clear is that they are in need of a special kind of healing. This is true regardless of whether the addicted spouse goes into recovery and gets better.

FORGIVENESS

Even though the addicted spouse has a disease and isn't fully responsible for his or her actions, the other spouse must still go through a process of forgiveness.

The key to understanding forgiveness is that it's literally a *selfish* act—it's something you do by yourself, for yourself. Forgiving another person doesn't change the other person; it only changes you because it allows you to let go of anger and resentment. Nor is forgiveness the result of something the other person does. Many spouses brood about how they want the addicted spouse to do something to "make it up to them," but the truth is that there is nothing an addicted spouse can do to make it up to the other spouse. Forgiveness is something you do because it makes *you* feel better; it's not something that the other person can merit.

Of all the precious things of which addiction can rob a family member, perhaps the saddest is the ability to love. The ability to love gets lost in all the anger and resentment. The thing that once made the soul soar is instead weighed down by a sack of bricks. Forgiveness is the process of *choosing* to toss aside the bricks, so as to be able to love again.

ENABLING IS DIFFERENT WITH SPOUSES

The strategy of avoiding enabling and allowing natural consequences is different with a spouse than it is with a child.

With children, you can hold over their head the consequence of not being able to live at home. But you can't simply threaten to kick a spouse out of the house if the spouse owns half the house.

If children have financial problems because of drugs or gambling, you can allow them to experience the natural consequences. But if your spouse loses a job or gambles away the rent money, you too are affected.

If a spouse drinks too much and throws up all over the living room sofa, you can't just say "too bad" . . . because it's also *your* sofa.

The point is that allowing natural consequences is much more complicated with a spouse than it is with a child, sibling, or other relative or friend. Whatever consequences you allow, they often affect you just as much. As a result, the advice to take care of yourself and the advice to avoid enabling come into conflict because taking care of yourself often means doing things that make the addict's life easier as well.

There's no simple solution to this dilemma. Spouses have to keep themselves safe and healthy and try to adapt the strategies for helping the addict as best they can. The key thing to remember is that self-caring and self-protective behavior is very important and that looking out for yourself is a good thing to do even if, in the short term, it might also appear to be enabling a spouse.

DEALING WITH YOUNG CHILDREN

One of the hardest things for spouses of addicts is dealing with young children living at home. Children tend to experience the same sorts of emotions as any other family member, but if they are young, they may have even more difficulty processing them.

When someone attempts to use CRAFT-style techniques with an addicted spouse, younger children can sometimes feel very upset. They experience the addicted spouse as mean, unloving, and rejecting of them. They often want the other spouse to "come to their rescue" and rebuke the addicted spouse, thus proving that at least one parental figure still loves them. And yet the other spouse is responding to the addicted spouse with positive communication and positive reinforcement! This suggests to the children that the other spouse is somehow on the addicted spouse's side and doesn't understand how they are being hurt.

Again, there's no perfect solution to this problem.

It can be helpful to explain to younger children that the addicted spouse has a disease. One way to describe it is that the addicted spouse has an "allergy." Many young children understand the concept of an allergy; they may have a friend at their school with a peanut allergy, for instance. They may be able to conceptualize that the addicted spouse has an allergy to alcohol or drugs and that this explains the spouse's behavior.

The advantage of this approach is that the children may be able to separate the behavior from the person and not feel so strongly that the addicted spouse's behavior is directed at them. Children may be less upset if they understand that the addicted spouse's behavior is being caused by a substance and is not a reaction to the children themselves. They may also experience less shame and guilt. (Children often blame themselves for a parent's addictive behavior because they can't think of any other cause, so giving them another cause can absolve them and make them feel less guilty.)

Obviously, it's important to hear out children's feelings and reassure them that you love them and understand what they're going through. To the extent that they can understand it, you can explain the techniques you're using and their purpose, so the children won't feel so betrayed.

DEALING WITH OLDER CHILDREN

As children get older, it can be very helpful for them to talk to a therapist about their feelings, especially one who has training in addiction and experience working with young people. As discussed in Chapter 13, support groups such as Alateen and Narateen can also be valuable.

It's not uncommon for adolescent children growing up with an addicted parent to make friends with other children in the same situation. This gives them someone to talk to who can understand their problems, and they may be willing to invite such children to their home (whereas they may avoid inviting other friends for fear that the parent will embarrass them). If a small group of such children get to know each other, the result can be a helpful, informal type of group therapy.

The most common problem children of addicted parents face is that the addict is simply missing in action as a parent. Children have to grow up without the guidance and support they would ordinarily receive. Worse, the roles are often reversed, and teenage children end up parenting their mother or father—taking care of their physical needs, understanding their problems, and giving them emotional support. In effect, the addict plays the role of the immature adolescent in the family, and the "real" adolescent is forced to play the role of adult.

Teenagers react to this situation in different ways. Some act out destructively—as though they're determined to reclaim their role and "out-adolescent" the parent. Some become depressed because they can't handle the emotional demands placed on them. Some grow up fast and become emotionally mature well beyond their years.

For spouses of an addict, the most important thing is to communicate love to the children and try to understand what they're going through. It's normal to be obsessed with the spouse and with your own feelings, but it's important to remember that children need attention and support no matter how distracting the spouse's behavior is.

16

Dealing with a Parent
Who Is an Addict

There are two kinds of older people who suffer from addiction: people who have been addicted for decades and have survived to an old age and late-onset addicts who first developed a problem in middle age or as senior citizens. These two types pose different problems for their adult children.

LATE-ONSET ADDICTS

Most people don't imagine senior citizens as alcoholics or drug addicts, but statistically it's surprisingly common. While addiction still occurs less frequently among seniors than among young people, U.S. government figures show that misuse of alcohol and prescription drugs by the elderly is one of the fastest-growing health problems in the country and affects as many as 17 percent of people over age 60.

Problem drinking by older women has become a significant issue recently. One study found that among women over 60 in the United States, binge drinking increased at an average rate of 3.7 percent per year between 1997 and 2014.

One cause of late-onset addiction is that people who have an underlying susceptibility may be triggered to begin actively abusing substances by the stressful changes that occur to them as senior citizens.

These include major and often deeply troubling life events such as retirement, mental or physical decline, financial worries, disease, social isolation, having to sell one's home or move into an assisted living facility, the death of a spouse or of close friends, and so on. These can lead to depression, which can in turn make addiction more likely to develop.

Sadly, even if an older adult begins to suffer from an addiction, children and other family members are often slow to pick up on what's going on. That's especially true where parents live alone because it's easier for them to hide the symptoms than it would be for a spouse or a child living at home. It can also be true if the older person has a history of moderate to heavy drinking in the past because drinking will seem "normal" to the children and it's difficult for them to realize that a bad habit has evolved into something more serious.

A major reason elderly addiction often goes undetected is that the most common symptoms frequently mirror those of old age itself. Seniors who are abusing substances may exhibit memory lapses, depression, sleep problems, chronic pain, loss of interest in former activities, and similar issues—and yet family members who would be highly suspicious of such developments in a younger person will often chalk them up in an older person to old age or the onset of dementia. Even medical personnel tend to be slow to pick up on the signs of elderly substance abuse.

In addition, older people are often retired and have fewer life responsibilities, so it's not as obvious when addiction gets in the way of their accomplishing things. The signs may be further masked by the fact that senior citizens usually require less alcohol to get "high," and so their drinking may appear relatively moderate—and older people often have lots of pills to take, so it can be harder to perceive that they're being abused.

The good news is that, in general, senior citizens respond to addiction treatment every bit as well as younger people do, so if it's possible to get them into a treatment program, there's a lot of hope.

But there are special challenges for children who are attempting to get an older person into treatment.

Parents who are dealing with an addicted child are at least used to taking charge of the child's life and helping to guide their son or daughter. And spouses usually have long experience helping each other in a variety of situations. But many children feel very awkward about telling their parents that they have a major life problem and need to get help.

Parents who don't want to acknowledge their addiction can be very effective at playing on this sensitivity and making their children who try to confront them feel ungrateful and callous. Some addicted parents have also been known to threaten children—directly or indirectly—with the loss of an inheritance if they keep talking about the issue.

Children who are already burdened with a lot of caretaking responsibilities for an older parent may feel that trying to deal with the addiction as well is overwhelming—and may even alienate the parent and limit their ability to care for the parent's needs in other ways.

And while it can be very hard for two parents to present a united front with an addicted child, it can be even more difficult to corral a number of siblings into being on the same page, especially if they don't live close by and see each other all the time. This can make it easy for a parent to play one sibling off another.

In addition, sometimes a sibling will be in denial about the problem. In the case of alcoholics, this can often be expressed with an attitude of "They're old; what difference does it make? Let them drink and have a good time." (Of course, older addicts are *not* having a good time, and the entire family is missing out on what could be very meaningful interactions.)

It can often be useful for siblings to meet with an addiction counselor who can help them work together and suggest ways to nudge the addicted parent toward acknowledging the problem and getting help.

CHILDREN OF LONG-TERM ADDICTS

If a person is a long-term addict rather than a late-onset addict, then the chances are significant that his or her children grew up with a parent who was in active addiction at least part of the time and have been considerably damaged in a number of ways by the experience. As a result, it can be a key priority for such children to get help for their own emotional issues.

It's likely that such children won't be able to be of much assistance to their parent unless they first come to terms with the psychological challenges caused by their own upbringing. (In fact, many children of addicted parents don't even want to help their parent. They are too angry and resentful.)

In 1983, psychologist Janet Woititz published a book called *Adult Children of Alcoholics,* which suggested that people who grew up with an alcoholic parent tend to have certain personality traits that make it difficult for them to function in the world. The book spawned a number of other books on the topic, and, as we've mentioned, there is also a popular support group based on the Twelve-Step model called Adult Children of Alcoholics.

According to Woititz, adult children of alcoholics often have these characteristics:

- They are impulsive and have difficulty following through on projects.
- They lie unnecessarily.
- They take themselves very seriously and judge themselves harshly.
- They have difficulty having fun.
- They have difficulty with intimate relationships.
- They overreact to changes over which they have no control.
- They constantly seek approval.
- They feel different from other people.
- They are either highly responsible or highly irresponsible.
- They are extremely loyal, even when loyalty is undeserved.
- Not having grown up in a normal household, they often have to guess at what "normal" behavior is.

Two observations can be made about this theory. The first is that, happily, not all children of alcoholics (or addicts in general) exhibit these traits. In fact, some children of addicts manage to escape relatively unscathed. This can be particularly true if the parent became addicted after the child was already a teenager, if the parent was not violent or abusive, or if the nonaddicted parent was psychologically healthy and able to provide an atmosphere of love and support.

The second observation is that these problems tend to result from having a parent who, because of the addiction, was distant, preoccupied, self-centered, and antagonistic and generally behaved in an uncaring and unloving manner. But these sorts of negative parental behaviors can result from many causes *other* than addiction. For instance, they can be the result of poverty and stress, other types of mental illness, an abusive personality, the fact that the parent didn't want the child and resented being a caregiver, or other life problems that the parent dealt with by taking them out on the child. Many children who were raised in foster care or who were adopted from troubled homes or orphanages have similar issues.

Thus, while the book and the support group are called Adult Children of Alcoholics, the problems they deal with tend to be more the result of growing up in a dysfunctional family, regardless of the cause. In actual practice, the support group often tends to attract and welcome people who grew up in family situations that were dysfunctional even if addiction played little or no role in the problem.

That said, families with an addict are almost by definition dysfunctional, and it's hard to overestimate the effect on a child of growing up with an addicted parent. Even adult children who feel and seem "normal" may still bear the scars and have simply found ways to adapt to them.

III

KEEPING AN ADDICT OUT OF TROUBLE

17

Can an Employee Be Fired for Having an Addiction?

You might be surprised to learn that an employee can't always be fired just for being an addict. A number of laws provide workplace protections for people who suffer from an addiction.

That doesn't mean that addicts can *never* be fired. They can—especially if the addiction results in poor work performance. But it's often more complicated than you might think.

This chapter will discuss the most important legal rules regarding addiction and employment in the United States. Other countries have different laws, although there are often a number of similarities. You can find help with other countries' laws in the Resources at the back of the book.

It's important to note that this book is not legal advice. If you have any questions, you should speak to an employment lawyer who can analyze how the law applies to your specific situation. Some suggestions for finding such a lawyer appear at the end of this chapter.

THE AMERICANS WITH DISABILITIES ACT

The most important U.S. law affecting addiction in the workplace is the Americans with Disabilities Act, often called the ADA. This federal law says that employers cannot harass or otherwise discriminate against employees because of a disability. It also says that employers must make reasonable accommodations to help disabled workers to perform their job duties. Violations of the ADA by an employer are illegal, and the employee can sue.

You might or might not want to contemplate actually bringing a lawsuit, but regardless of whether you do, it's important to know your legal rights. The more you understand the rules, the better you can advocate for yourself or a family member, and the stronger your negotiating position. Most employers really do want to do the right thing and follow the law, and all employers worry about the legal consequences of disobeying it.

You're probably wondering, "Is an addiction a disability?" Generally, yes. The ADA defines a disability as a physical or mental impairment that substantially limits a major life activity. Major life activities include thinking, communicating, concentrating, working, caring for oneself, and having normal brain and neurological functioning.

There's generally no question that addiction is a physical or mental impairment. Most of the time, it's also fairly obvious that it substantially limits a major life activity. Therefore, in most cases, addiction qualifies as a disability.

Importantly, the law says that an employee who had an addiction-related disability at some point in the past, but is now in recovery, is still considered to have a disability.

Since addiction is a disability, an employer cannot harass, punish, or otherwise discriminate against an employee for having it. For instance, a boss cannot fire or demote someone simply for being an alcoholic or in recovery from a drug problem. A boss also can't favor one worker over another for a promotion due to the fact of an addiction. And a boss cannot tolerate a workplace environment in which coworkers harass someone over a past or present addiction issue.

But that said, a boss *can* fire or discipline employees if their work performance isn't good enough—even if the reason the performance isn't good enough is the addiction.

Of course, very often an addiction causes work performance to suffer, so an employer may be in the right in disciplining an employee anyway. However, employers have to be extremely careful to base any disciplinary action on a documented history of poor performance, as opposed to the mere fact of an addiction. As long as an employee is fulfilling the requirements of the job, a boss can get into big trouble for taking the fact of an addiction into account.

While it's certainly possible for an addicted employee to bring a discrimination lawsuit, in the real world this is often made more difficult by the stigma of addiction. Employees are usually in a stronger position to win a case—or to otherwise advocate for their rights—if one or more of the following is true:

- It's clear that the employee's work performance was very good, or at least wasn't affected by the addiction (for instance, the employee's performance evaluations were similar before and after the addiction started).
- The discrimination was based on a history of addiction rather than on an active addiction in the present—so there's no possibility that the employee's current work performance was affected.
- The employee was proactive in addressing his or her problem and quickly seeking help.
- The employer made derogatory comments about addicts in general or otherwise demonstrated a bias against addiction rather than focusing solely on work performance.

Reasonable Accommodation

The ADA says that employers are required to "reasonably accommodate" disabled employees if doing so will enable them to adequately perform their job.

It's not always clear what this means in the case of an addiction, but some judges have decided that it can include giving employees a leave of absence to attend rehab or altering their work schedule so they can attend Alcoholics Anonymous or other meetings.

However, judges have generally ruled that an employer doesn't have to *pay* for rehab if it's not covered by the employee's health insurance. And they have sometimes allowed employers to refuse to provide a leave of absence if the employer can show that it's unlikely to work—for instance, if the employee has repeatedly dropped out of rehab and relapsed in the past.

Exceptions to the ADA

The ADA creates broad rules that help addicts, but it also contains a number of important exceptions.

For instance, the law makes an important distinction between alcoholics and drug addicts. The law covers alcoholics regardless of whether they are currently abusing alcohol or are in treatment or recovery. However, while the law covers drug addicts *in recovery*, it doesn't cover drug addicts who are currently using drugs illegally.

That means, for instance, that an employee who is currently using heroin can be fired for that reason alone—even if the person would otherwise be protected by the ADA as an addict with a disability.

It's not always clear whether a person is "currently" using drugs. Most judges have ruled that people are currently using drugs if they fail a drug test or if they were using drugs regularly in the past weeks or months. As a result, a person might still be considered a "current" drug user even if he or she very recently went into rehab.

Also, the exception applies only to people who are currently using drugs *illegally*. It's possible that an addict might be abusing opioids, for instance, but not doing so illegally because at the moment he or she has a prescription.

Other exceptions to the ADA include:

- The law doesn't apply to small businesses—those with fewer than 15 employees.
- Process addictions might not count under the ADA. The law specifically excludes compulsive gambling and sexual behavior disorders, and it might be hard to prove that other types of process addictions qualify as disabilities.
- The ADA doesn't apply to federal employees—although another law called the Rehabilitation Act *does* apply to federal workers and says much the same thing.
- The ADA allows employers to adopt a number of workplace rules related to drugs and alcohol. For instance, an employer can prohibit the presence of alcohol or illegal drugs in the workplace. An employer can also prohibit employees from being under the influence of alcohol or illegal drugs while they're at work and can fire or discipline them if they are.
- There are exceptions for certain safety-sensitive jobs. The ADA doesn't preempt other laws concerning addicts who work as law enforcement officers, airline pilots, truck drivers, or railroad engineers, as well as those who work in nuclear plants, on federal contracts, or in certain military operations.

Drug Tests

Since the ADA doesn't protect employees who are currently using drugs illegally, employers typically have free rein to force workers to take tests to see if they're using illegal drugs.

However, some types of tests may reveal other medical information in addition to whether the person is using illegal drugs. These types of tests may be illegal.

In general, employers may not ask workers if they are currently taking drugs *legally* (such as painkillers for which they have a prescription). However, if an employee flunks a drug test, the employer may ask if he or she is taking any prescription drugs that could have influenced the result.

Alcohol tests are more restricted. Although the law is a bit unclear, the general rule is that employees can't be tested randomly for alcohol. They can be tested only if the employer has a reasonable suspicion that a particular employee is drunk at work or that alcohol use is impairing the employee's performance or creating a safety problem.

Job Applicants

The ADA provides protection not only to employees but also to job applicants.

For instance, under the ADA an employer generally cannot ask job applicants if they are alcoholics or drug addicts or if they have ever attended a rehab program.

An employer can ask about prior drug or alcohol use, but not in a way that might reveal whether the person has an addiction. So, for instance, an employer can ask if an applicant drinks or has ever used illegal drugs, but it cannot ask how often or how much or for how long.

Employers can give drug tests to job applicants, but not alcohol tests.

Once an employer has chosen a candidate for a job, it can make a job offer that is conditional on finding out further information about disabilities. At this point, the employer can ask about addiction-related issues and can give an alcohol test. However, the employer still cannot discriminate—which means that it must give the candidate the position unless the answers to the disability questions indicate that he or she wouldn't be able to perform the essential functions of the job, even with a reasonable accommodation.

OTHER DISABILITY PROTECTIONS

Many U.S. states have their own laws against disability discrimination. Most of these are similar to the ADA, but there can be differences that are helpful to workers. For instance, some state laws may apply to small businesses with fewer than 15 employees.

In addition to state laws, some union agreements may also offer protections to workers with an addiction. This is especially true in the area of drug testing.

THE FAMILY AND MEDICAL LEAVE ACT

Another important U.S. law is the federal Family and Medical Leave Act, or FMLA, which allows employees to take protected job leave if they have a serious medical issue or if they are taking care of a family member with such an issue. In many cases, people receiving addiction treatment (or who have a family member who is receiving treatment) qualify for leave.

The FMLA applies to all government employees. It also applies to private employees if (1) the employee has worked for the employer for at least a year, (2) the employee has worked at least 1,250 hours during the last year, and (3) the employer has at least 50 people working at the employee's location or within 75 miles of it.

The FMLA says that employees can take up to 12 weeks of protected leave per year to deal with their own or a family member's serious medical condition. Generally, addiction qualifies as a serious medical condition. "Protected leave" means that employees must be reinstated in their old job when they return or given a similar job with equal pay.

In many cases, employees can take "intermittent leave," meaning they can be absent from the workplace for a day or even a few hours at a time rather than taking their leave all at once. This can be very helpful if an addict needs to attend support-group meetings, therapy sessions, outpatient treatment, and so on.

There are some important restrictions, however. For instance, employees can take FMLA leave only if they are in (or their family member is in) a form of treatment that is provided or recommended by a health care provider. Employees can't take protected leave simply because they are addicted or are abusing substances.

While an employer can't fire someone for taking FMLA leave, employers can still fire someone for violating an established workplace policy regarding illegal drugs—even if they otherwise qualify for FMLA leave.

Also, employees must usually provide certain types of advance notice to qualify for FMLA leave. This can be tricky in the case of addiction because many people wind up in treatment as a result of a surprise intervention or a sudden medical crisis, with the result that providing advance notice can be difficult.

Finally, employers aren't required to pay employees their salary while they take FMLA leave, and in practice very few do.

About a dozen U.S. states have their own family and medical leave laws. These are important because they sometimes cover people who don't qualify for coverage under the federal law (for instance, because they haven't worked for the employer long enough or because the employer doesn't have enough employees). In addition, some state laws provide for partially paid family and medical leave.

"LAST CHANCE" AGREEMENTS

Many employers want to be compassionate toward good workers who are facing up to their addiction problems and seeking treatment. In many cases, these employers could legally fire the employee for poor performance, but they want to give the person one last chance to straighten out and keep the job.

The result is a written contract that is commonly known as a "last-chance agreement." In it, the employee promises to go to treatment and follow a program of recovery and acknowledges that he or she can be fired immediately if there's a slip-up.

Ideally, the agreement should provide answers to a number of questions about how the deal will work. For instance:

- Who will pay for the treatment? Will it be covered by the employee's health insurance at work?
- If the employee will miss work due to treatment, will this be considered family and medical leave, sick leave, vacation, personal leave, or some combination?
- Can the company monitor the employee's participation in the treatment program?

- After the employee returns to work, will the company perform unannounced drug or alcohol tests?
- Does the company have a right to receive medical information from the employee's doctors? If so, what must the employee do to waive his or her medical privacy rights? What happens if the employee's substance-abuse treatment overlaps with treatment for some other medical problem that the company doesn't have a right to know about?
- What constitutes a slip-up for which the employee can be fired? Can the employee be terminated for missing a therapy appointment, for instance, or only if he or she relapses?

A big issue with last-chance agreements is that it might be illegal for a company to ask an employee to sign one unless it can document that the employee's substance abuse problem has actually created problems at work.

For example, an assistant fire chief in Lima, Ohio, became addicted to opioids following his treatment for kidney stones. His painkiller addiction grew into a heroin addiction, and he voluntarily checked into a rehab facility. While he was in rehab, he got a visit from the fire chief, who told him he'd have to sign a last-chance agreement to avoid being fired.

But a state appeals court ruled this could be illegal disability discrimination. Because the employee had no prior performance issues, the fire chief's order suggested that he was being punished merely for his status as a recovering addict, rather than for any actual workplace problems that he had caused.

On the other hand, a federal appeals court in Philadelphia decided that a freight company had a right to force a driver to sign a last-chance agreement after he took medical leave to go to an alcohol rehab program, despite a clean work record in the past. The court said that this was okay because a truck driver who consumes alcohol at work could pose a serious and immediate risk of injury.

Employers also can't discriminate in the way they *enforce* last-chance agreements. For example, an employee who signed such an agreement and was fired after a brief slip-up could potentially sue for discrimination if the employer had signed similar agreements with other employees in the past and had "forgiven" them despite repeated relapses.

FILING A COMPLAINT

The Equal Employment Opportunity Commission, or EEOC, is the federal agency that enforces discrimination laws in the United States. Generally, the first step for employees in claiming that an employer violated the ADA is to file a complaint, or "charge," with the EEOC. Employees typically must do this before they can bring a private lawsuit.

If the EEOC thinks that an employee has a good case and that the case will help it to establish an important legal precedent, it can bring a discrimination lawsuit on the employee's behalf. This is good news for the employee because it means that he or she doesn't have to pay for a lawyer. However, it's unusual.

Sometimes the EEOC will encourage the two sides to resolve their dispute through voluntary mediation.

Otherwise, or if the mediation doesn't work, the EEOC will give the employee a "right to sue" letter. This letter means that the employee can bring a private lawsuit.

You can learn more about the EEOC's charge system at *www.eeoc.gov/employees/charge.cfm*.

Most states have an agency similar to the EEOC that enforces the state's own discrimination laws. The process is usually very similar. In general, employees who believe that an employer has violated both state and federal laws can file with the state agency, and the state agency will notify the EEOC; it's not necessary to file two separate complaints.

FINDING A LAWYER

Employees who want to file a private lawsuit—or just generally want to consult with someone about their legal rights—should try to find a lawyer who specializes in employment law. Most employment lawyers further specialize in representing either employees or employers, so it's best to find one who specializes in representing employees.

There are a number of find-a-lawyer services available—in the United States, some of the most reputable are operated by state bar associations—but these won't necessarily lead you to the most accomplished and successful attorneys. Lawyers who sign up for these services are often younger and less experienced attorneys who are looking for work. More accomplished specialists tend to get cases through other means, such as referrals from past clients and from other lawyers who are in general practice or in different specialties.

So, a good approach is to look for lawyers who have a successful track record in similar cases. For instance, in the United States there's a national professional organization of attorneys dedicated to representing employees in workplace lawsuits, called the National Employment Lawyers Association. You can search for members by city and state (as well as for affiliated members in Canada and Mexico) at *http://exchange. nela.org/memberdirectory/findalawyer.*

Another approach is to search the Internet for news articles about workplace disputes involving addiction in your area. You might turn up articles about recent cases, which will tell you the name of the lawyer who represented the employee. You might also find articles about the issue in general, which will quote local lawyers. Presumably, the reporter went to some effort to find credible, knowledgeable lawyers to interview, and you can piggyback on the reporter's research rather than reinventing the wheel.

Lawyers with a specialty practice tend to know other lawyers in the same field and generally have a sense of who the best ones are. If you find a highly credible lawyer with a relevant background who's somewhat outside your geographic area, you could call his or her office and ask for a referral to someone local. This might not work, but it sometimes does. Lawyers are often happy to refer potential clients to colleagues in a different locale because they hope they'll someday get a similar referral in return.

18

Drug Courts and Other Ways to Keep an Addict Out of Jail

I t's not surprising that addicts often get into trouble with the law. Typical criminal charges include drug possession, drug dealing, driving under the influence, public drunkenness, property crimes designed to obtain money for drugs, and so on.

In response, the United States and many other countries have created specialized "drug courts" that are designed to get addicts into treatment rather than simply putting them behind bars. Instead of going to jail, being put on probation, or facing some other traditional form of criminal punishment, the addict is given the option of attending a treatment program. The addict's attendance at the program and success at staying clean and sober (or at least out of further trouble with the law) are monitored by the court. Addicts who successfully complete the program get to go free, and the other criminal consequences are waived or extremely limited.

The first drug court was an experiment conducted in Miami, Florida, in 1989. Today there are more than 3,000 such programs across the United States, according to the National Association of Drug Court Professionals. There are even specialized court programs for alcoholics, for people with gambling problems, for juvenile addicts, and for young offenders whose parents have an addiction.

Drug court programs have also been established in Australia, Belgium, Bermuda, Brazil, Canada, Chile, England, Ireland, Jamaica,

Mauritius, Mexico, New Zealand, Northern Ireland, Norway, Scotland, Suriname, and Wales.

The idea behind these programs is that addicts don't commit crimes because they have a moral failing; they commit crimes because they have a disease. If the justice system can treat the disease, it can prevent future crimes and reduce the overall cost to society—much more effectively than jail time will.

These programs are often called diversionary programs, since the goal is to divert people away from the standard criminal justice system.

Family members are often horrified when an addicted family member gets arrested. However, in some cases, an arrest can mean that the justice system gains leverage to get the addict into treatment—which is exactly what the family had been trying unsuccessfully to do all along.

When possible, therefore, it's usually a good idea for a family to try to steer an addict who has been arrested into a drug-court program.

HOW IT WORKS

This chapter will look at how drug-court programs operate in the United States. Other countries' programs tend to be similar, but the specifics may vary. (More information about programs in other countries can be found in the Resources at the back of the book.)

Generally in the United States, the first three steps in a drug-court program are evaluation, screening, and assessment. Many people get these three confused because they sound like similar things, but they are actually separate steps in the process.

Evaluation

Evaluation means determining whether the addict is eligible for the program in the first place. Not everyone who commits a crime is eligible for drug court. Usually, a court will set specific guidelines for who is eligible, based on the nature of the crime and the person's criminal record.

Some courts limit eligible crimes to nonviolent offenses, or to probation revocation, or to crimes specifically related to substances, such as drug possession or drunk driving. As for the person's record, some courts will take only first-time offenders. Some will accept repeat offenders, but this may depend on the nature of the prior offense or whether the person previously served jail time.

The evaluation is often performed by the prosecutor and the judge, although the defendant's lawyer might be able to participate.

Screening

Assuming a person is legally eligible for drug court, the next step is screening, which is where the court determines whether it's likely that the person would benefit from the program. Usually this means determining whether the person is an addict and whether the addiction can be treated with the resources that the court has available. For example, if the person has a serious mental health issue in addition to addiction, and that issue would likely interfere with the addiction treatment, the person might not pass the screening. (Some courts have other types of diversionary programs for people with serious mental health issues, and the person might be referred to that type of program instead.)

Other personnel may get involved at the screening stage, including treatment professionals and the local health department.

Some courts have limited funding and may restrict their program to what they consider the most serious cases. For instance, some programs will admit people who are addicted to heroin or methamphetamine, but not people who abuse alcohol or marijuana.

Assessment

Defendants who pass both the evaluation and the screening are accepted into the drug-court program. At this point they receive an assessment, which is a more detailed examination of their treatment needs conducted by professionals with specialized training. The assessment is then used to create an individualized treatment plan. The treatment plan specifies what activities defendants must participate in and for how long, as well as the consequences if they fail to show up or get into further trouble.

A few courts skip the screening stage and conduct a full assessment before deciding whether to accept someone into the program. This can be helpful in some cases. A problem, though, is that an assessment requires addicts to disclose a great deal more about their history and condition than they would have to in a simple screening. Some addicts are understandably reluctant to make such a full disclosure to people in the justice system before they know for certain whether they will be accepted into the program.

Some drug courts simply provide addiction treatment services, along with drug testing and other measures to monitor compliance. But other programs are more robust and partner with other agencies to provide a wider range of services to help addicts get back on their feet and to reintegrate them into the community. These services can include help in finding jobs, housing, transportation, and health care, as well as financial counseling, GED (high school equivalency) and ESL (English as a second language) classes, and civil legal assistance programs.

MUST YOU PLEAD GUILTY?

There are two types of drug-court arrangements. In the first type, the addict enters the program without having to enter a plea at all. If the addict successfully completes the program, the charges are simply dropped. If the addict doesn't successfully complete the program, the case goes back to criminal court for prosecution.

In the second type, the addict must plead guilty to the charges. The plea is entered, but the sentencing is deferred or suspended. If the addict successfully completes the program, the sentence is waived, and in some cases the offense may be expunged from the person's record. If the addict doesn't successfully complete the program, the case goes back to criminal court and a sentence is imposed based on the guilty plea.

When drug courts first began to be popular in the 1990s, they were almost always of the first type. The reason is that drug courts were initially intended solely for first-time offenders charged with very minor offenses. The overriding goal was to get these people into treatment before they became more serious criminals, and the justice system wasn't deeply concerned about its ability to prosecute people for first-time public intoxication, for example.

But as drug courts showed success, they began to be expanded and applied to repeat offenders and people charged with more serious crimes. All of a sudden, the justice system *did* have an interest in prosecuting drug-court defendants fully if they failed to complete a treatment program. However, if prosecutors had to wait for months to find out if an addict would succeed at recovery before they could go to trial, it could become a lot harder to get a conviction. Evidence could be lost, witnesses' memories could fade, and so on. For this reason, many prosecutors insisted that drug courts adopt the second type of arrangement, so they could be sure of having a conviction if the addict didn't complete treatment.

Today a single drug court may operate using both systems, with the necessity of pleading guilty depending on the nature of the charges and the defendant's record.

Any addict considering going into a drug-court program should be aware of whether a guilty plea will be required and whether the charges will be expunged from his or her record if treatment is successful. A criminal defense lawyer may be able to explain the possible consequences of a conviction in later life, including what it may mean for employment, government benefits, immigration, and any future criminal charges.

ARE THE PROGRAMS SUCCESSFUL?

There are very few statistics as to exactly how successful drug-court programs are in getting addicts well, although anything that gets large numbers of addicts into treatment can't help being a good thing. Many drug-court studies have been conducted by the justice system, and these tend to focus on the effect of the programs on the system itself rather than on clinical outcomes. For instance, the U.S. Department of Justice has published figures showing that people who go through drug-court programs often have dramatically lower recidivism rates than other defendants, meaning that they're much less likely to get into further trouble with the law. While that doesn't necessarily prove that they have overcome their addiction, it suggests that the programs have helped many people get their lives back on track in a number of ways.

Nevertheless, not everyone likes drug courts. Some people argue that the courts fill up treatment programs with people who are there not because they want to be, but because they are simply trying to avoid jail, and thus funding is diverted from voluntary programs that might have a better chance of success. Some criminal defense lawyers complain that the programs encourage police to arrest apparent addicts for negligible crimes and then pressure them to plead guilty before a lawyer can properly investigate the facts and decide whether the case can be won at trial.

Furthermore, some advocates for drug legalization or decriminalization argue that the drug-court system, while compassionate, still perpetuates the idea that drug use is a criminal justice problem rather than a public health issue—and they argue that judges and prosecutors are not the best-trained people to be making decisions about mental health treatment.

POLICE INITIATIVES TO HELP ADDICTS

In some parts of the United States, it's not the court system but the police who are trying to replace jail time with treatment for addicts.

In 2015, the police department in Gloucester, Massachusetts, started a program in which people who were using opioids or other drugs could simply go to a police station and ask for help and the police would guide them into treatment. The police department promised that anyone who went to a station and asked for help would not be charged with a crime. Even if people arrived at a station with drugs on them, the police would dispose of the drugs and no charges would be filed.

By most measures the program was a success. In the first year, about 400 people showed up at a station and were guided into treatment. There was only one overdose death in Gloucester during that year, compared to five the previous year. Drug crime in the city declined 27 percent, and property crimes such as burglary and shoplifting (often associated with people trying to get money for drugs) declined as well. An independent study showed that 60 percent of program participants had managed to avoid relapse. What's more, the department said that the cost of sending people to treatment was about one-quarter that of processing them through the court system.

Within a little over a year, some 160 other police departments across the country had created similar programs.

These initiatives often have broad community support. The one group that has occasionally been suspicious of them, however, is prosecutors, in part because some prosecutors believe that the police are infringing on their turf by making decisions about whether to charge someone with a crime.

William Fitzpatrick, chairman of the National District Attorneys Association, called police programs to help addicts "a really stupid idea." He argued that such programs are illegal because police officers don't have a right to grant people immunity and that drug courts are preferable to police amnesty programs because the threat of prosecution is necessary to get addicts to stick to a treatment regimen.

But these sentiments are not universal. Many prosecutors strongly support such police initiatives. In fact, a 2016 law review article considered 112 police amnesty programs that had been established in the previous 15 months and noted that not a single district attorney had taken any action to suspend such a program, even though they could have done so.

Interestingly, the New Jersey Supreme Court has ruled that if a person voluntarily turns over illegal drugs to police without being asked, this evidence can't be used in a prosecution for drug possession because doing so would violate the right against self-incrimination under the Fifth Amendment to the U.S. Constitution. The ruling isn't binding outside New Jersey, but it's still significant because it suggests that prosecutors might be wrong when they say that they have the authority to decide whether to prosecute such cases—under the U.S. Constitution, they might not.

19

Using Civil Commitment to Keep an Addict Safe

In most U.S. states and a number of other countries, a family member can go to court and ask that an addict who is a danger to himself or others be sent involuntarily to a treatment facility. This is usually called civil commitment.

Civil commitment is an extreme measure, and it's typically an unpleasant experience for all concerned. The addict may be arrested and brought into court, where family members may have to testify against him or her. The length of the commitment can be anywhere from a brief sobering-up period to a year in a locked facility. The commitment facilities themselves are often bare-bones at best, and treatment may be minimal.

Nevertheless, civil commitment is an important option for many families, for two reasons. The first is that it may be the best approach when addicts are truly a danger to themselves—when they are refusing help, engaging in highly reckless behavior, or suicidal—and the family has tried everything else and simply wants to make sure that the person stays alive for the near future. It can be a blessing to know that an addict will be locked up somewhere safe, and it can give the family time to come up with other options (and give the addict time to reflect on his or her situation).

The second advantage of civil commitment is that it can be used as a bargaining chip. If a family makes a credible threat to have an addict civilly committed, the addict might choose instead to go into some other form of voluntary treatment that is less bleak and harsh.

Of course, addicts typically react very negatively to the idea of being arrested and locked up, at least at first. The resulting sense of betrayal and lack of trust toward the family members responsible is something that has to be factored into the equation.

This chapter will provide an overview of how civil commitment works in the United States. (Information for other countries can be found in the Resources at the back of the book.) However, even within the United States, the rules vary considerably from state to state, and you'll want to consult a lawyer or court official if you're thinking seriously of using civil commitment.

WHERE IT CAME FROM

Back in 1962, the U.S. Supreme Court ruled that it was unconstitutional for the government to make it a crime to be an addict. Importantly, the court recognized that addiction is a disease, and it said it would be "cruel and unusual punishment" to put people in jail just because they had a disease. The court said a person could still be prosecuted for a specific act, such as possessing or using illegal drugs, but addiction by itself couldn't be a crime.

However, the court went on to say that a state could involuntarily commit an addict for treatment in certain situations. This would be *civil* (as opposed to criminal) commitment.

Civil commitment programs have been around in the United States since the 1800s, but at the beginning they were generally used only for other types of mental illness. After the 1962 decision, however, more states began to expand their civil commitment programs to include addiction. Today more than 30 states and the District of Columbia have laws that specifically allow for civil commitment of addicts.

According to a 2015 study, civil commitment for addiction is used most frequently in Arkansas, Colorado, Florida, Hawaii, Massachusetts, Minnesota, Missouri, Montana, South Carolina, South Dakota, Texas, Washington, West Virginia, and Wisconsin.

It is used less frequently in Alaska, Connecticut, Delaware, Georgia, Indiana, Iowa, Kansas, Kentucky, Louisiana, Maine, Mississippi, North Carolina, North Dakota, Ohio, Oklahoma, Rhode Island, Tennessee, Utah, and the District of Columbia.

In the remaining 18 states, civil commitment for addiction is largely nonexistent, but it might theoretically be allowed under laws that cover mental illness but don't specifically mention substance abuse. Only seven states specifically prohibit civil commitment for addiction (Alabama, Arizona, Idaho, Illinois, Nevada, New Hampshire, and Wyoming).

State laws vary as to who is allowed to initiate a civil commitment proceeding. Most commonly, a claim can be brought by a family member, guardian, doctor, or police officer. Many states also allow a criminal court to refer a defendant for civil commitment proceedings.

WHAT MUST YOU PROVE?

The most common rule is that addicts can be involuntarily committed if they are gravely disabled or pose an imminent danger to themselves or others. "Gravely disabled" means that the person is incapable of obtaining the basic necessities of life. An "imminent" danger means that the risk of harm is real and specific and the harm could happen in the very near future.

Back in the 1800s and early 1900s, the standards for civil commitment were very loose. Generally, a family could commit someone for long periods simply by claiming that the person had a mental illness and needed treatment. As a result, many families that wanted to seize control of a relative's assets, or simply get an inconvenient family member out of the way, concocted a story about how the relative was in need of treatment.

Abuses such as these led to a tightening of standards. In 1964, the District of Columbia adopted the "gravely disabled or imminent danger" standard, and many states have now followed suit and adopted something very similar. However, some states still have looser requirements. For instance, Iowa allows commitment if an addict cannot make "responsible decisions" regarding treatment and is likely to cause "serious emotional injury" to family members.

The "gravely disabled or imminent danger" standard can be a significant stumbling block for families. For example, a family may be distraught because an addicted child is living hand to mouth, couch-surfing or occasionally homeless, out of communication, and acting extremely recklessly. But if the child is consistently able to find some sort of food and shelter and has never threatened to hurt anyone or commit suicide, it can be difficult to prove that he or she is gravely disabled or poses an imminent danger.

Whatever the state's standard, the Supreme Court ruled in 1979 that a family must provide evidence that is "clear and convincing." It's not enough merely to show that it's *likely* the addict meets the standard; a family has to provide proof that leaves little doubt about the matter. However, the evidence doesn't have to meet the traditional requirement of a criminal case, which is proof "beyond a reasonable doubt."

How do all these rules and standards play out in actual practice? The answer varies a great deal from state to state and, in fact, from case to case. Judges certainly want addicts to be cared for, but they're also understandably reluctant to lock people up and take away their freedom if they haven't committed a crime.

In practice, some judges will accept a doctor's letter stating that an addict meets the standard as sufficient evidence, unless the addict can somehow prove otherwise. Some judges will accept a letter from a psychologist, an addiction counselor, or another type of medical professional. Some will allow a commitment if the addict was recently treated for substance abuse on an emergency basis.

Some judges won't commit someone involuntarily unless the family can show that the addict refused a voluntary treatment plan that was practical and affordable.

Of course, some judges will simply accept a family member's testimony that the addict is out of control and needs help—particularly if the addict can't make a convincing case to the contrary.

WHAT'S THE PROCEDURE?

The procedure for a civil commitment case also varies from state to state, but commonly a family member will initiate the proceedings by filing a form with a court. If the addict doesn't come to court voluntarily to respond, the police may arrest him or her.

Because of past abuses in which family members were civilly committed based on little evidence, most states now require a formal hearing. Addicts may be given a lawyer to defend them and to argue against the need for commitment. Family members may have to testify about why they believe the addict is disabled or poses an imminent danger. Witnesses may be called, including friends, neighbors, and doctors. A judge will hear all the evidence and decide.

The good news for families is that, while some hearings can resemble a full-blown court trial, a lot of civil commitment proceedings are in reality much less dramatic. If the family is right and the addict really is gravely disabled, it's unlikely that he or she will have the ability to present a coherent and persuasive court case. Much of the time, it's immediately obvious to everyone that the addict needs to be committed, even if the person tries to argue to the contrary. And frequently an addict who is brought into court will simply agree to the commitment rather than fight it.

If a judge orders a commitment, it will be for a specific period of time. Each state has its own rules for the maximum length of a commitment, but a few weeks to a few months is common. Once committed, an addict will typically be given some form of treatment, which may include psychotherapy, drug therapy, or access to Twelve-Step meetings. (However, many state programs are cash-strapped and the level of treatment provided might not be ideal.)

Once the commitment period is over, the addict can go free, unless the family goes back to court and persuades a judge that further commitment is necessary. An addict doesn't have to prove that he or she is "better" to go free after the commitment period is up. Also, addicts cannot be ordered to continue treatment once they're no longer committed.

OUTPATIENT COMMITMENT

Recently a few states have begun experimenting with outpatient civil commitment. Rather than being sent to a locked facility, addicts may be given their freedom but ordered to go regularly to some form of outpatient treatment during the commitment period. If they refuse, or if they fail to show up for the treatment, they may then be committed to an inpatient facility.

It's generally easier to get someone committed to outpatient treatment because the standard is not as high. Rather than having to prove "gravely disabled or imminent danger," for instance, a family member might have to prove only that the addict needs treatment, is unlikely to go voluntarily, and without proper treatment is likely to *eventually* become gravely disabled.

Of course, outpatient treatment has its downsides. There's a greater risk that addicts will skip the treatment sessions and do harm to themselves before they can be locked up. Also, it's not as powerful a bargaining chip if the goal is to get the addict into a residential rehab program.

20

More Ways to Protect an Addict from Harm

This chapter will discuss some other ideas for protecting addicts (and their families) from serious harm, both before treatment and during recovery. They include ways to:

- Reverse an overdose
- Stop alcoholics from driving drunk
- Find out if an addict is using or relapsing
- Support recovering addicts in school
- Help when a recovering addict needs painkillers for medical reasons

Some of these techniques could be grouped under the heading "harm reduction." In general, harm reduction refers to efforts that are not specifically aimed at getting addicts to stop using, but instead are designed to reduce the collateral damage caused by using. On a societal scale, this could include initiatives such as needle exchange programs and safe injection sites, which are not intended to prevent the use of drugs but rather to stop overdoses and the spread of disease that can result from drug use. (Information on these types of programs can be found in the Resources at the back of the book.)

Harm reduction can be controversial because some people believe that reducing the potential harm associated with illegal drugs can cause more people to use them.

This sort of larger public policy debate is beyond the scope of this book. However, what's important to note is that family and friends can engage in their own form of "harm reduction" on a much smaller scale. And on this scale, the larger issues about harm reduction's merits simply don't apply. It's one thing to argue about the social value of needle exchange programs, but when the question is whether to save your child's life right now or to prevent your spouse from driving drunk with children in the car, there's no real question as to the right thing to do.

NARCAN

Narcan is a drug that can reverse an overdose of heroin or other opioids. If someone in your family is addicted to opioids, you should immediately obtain this drug and learn how to use it in an emergency. You should also try to get as many of the addict's family members and close friends as possible to do the same. It could save the person's life.

Narcan is the most common brand name for the drug naloxone. It's available as a generic medication, and it can have other brand names. It can be purchased without a prescription in all but a handful of U.S. states as well as in Australia, Canada, the United Kingdom, and a number of other countries.

Paramedics and other first responders typically carry Narcan, as do emergency rooms. A growing number of police officers carry Narcan as well, in case they respond to an overdose before paramedics arrive.

In the United States, a dose of Narcan typically retails for $100 to $150, but it is covered by most private insurance policies as well as Medicare and Medicaid, so most people have only a small copay. Narcan originally had to be injected with a needle, but since 2015 it has been available in a nasal spray version. The new version is much easier to use, and specialized training for family members is no longer required. However, you should still make sure you know exactly how to use it in advance; you don't want to be reading the instructions in an emergency. For example, if the person doesn't revive immediately after receiving a dose, it's recommended that you engage in a process called rescue breathing and then administer the drug a second time after several minutes. (More information about using Narcan can be found in the Resources at the back of the book.)

If you have a phone handy, always call emergency services (911 in the United States and Canada, 999 in the United Kingdom, 000 in Australia, and so forth) *before* administering Narcan. Paramedics have far more extensive resources at their disposal, and getting them to come quickly is the top priority. When speaking to an emergency operator, it's recommended that you give your location and say simply that the person is "unresponsive and not breathing." Sadly, because of the stigma surrounding addiction, saying that someone "had an overdose" may cause your case to be given a lower priority. Reporting that a person is unresponsive and not breathing tends to put the case at the top of the priority list.

Because people who have overdosed can choke if they vomit, you should try not to leave the person alone while waiting for help. If you must do so (to let paramedics in, for example), put the person on his or her left side with the face aimed downward and the upper leg tucked slightly toward the chest.

If the person does revive, you should be aware that Narcan doesn't just reverse the overdose—it reverses the entire effect of the drug. Thus, a person who has been given Narcan will experience sudden and acute withdrawal symptoms and may be very angry or irritable.

The effects of Narcan are short-lived. As a result, if a person is revived with Narcan but still has a significant amount of the drug in his or her system, the person may experience a second overdose once the Narcan wears off—requiring a second dose of Narcan. This is another reason it's important to call emergency services and get medical treatment as soon as possible.

Narcan should be stored at room temperature—between 15 and 25 degrees Celsius or 59 and 77 degrees Fahrenheit. While you might think it's a good idea to keep Narcan in your car, you should be aware that if your car is regularly exposed to lower or higher temperatures, the drug can lose its potency.

Narcan isn't magic. It doesn't always work, especially if an overdose isn't discovered right away. Also, higher-potency drugs such as fentanyl and carfentanil (which are sometimes cut with heroin or used in counterfeit prescription opioids) may be resistant to Narcan or may require multiple Narcan doses.

An alternative to Narcan is Evzio, which is not a nasal spray but a device that injects naloxone when held next to someone's thigh. One advantage of Evzio is that when you activate the device, it gives verbal instructions as to how to use it.

Some people have argued that the widespread use of Narcan has made opioid abusers more reckless because they think that overdoses are no longer fatal. But there's little hard evidence for this, and it's certainly no reason not to have a life-saving drug on hand.

Families should keep Narcan handy even if an opioid addict is in long-term recovery. In fact, Narcan can be even more critical in the event of a relapse than it is for a regular user. Regular heroin users, for instance, typically develop a tolerance for the drug and can gradually take larger and larger doses without experiencing respiratory failure. However, if a person takes the same dose after not having used heroin in a while, there's a much greater chance of an overdose.

CAR BREATH TESTS

It's possible to install a device in your car that will prevent it from starting until the driver passes an alcohol breath test. The driver must blow into a tube, and the engine will be blocked unless the driver's blood alcohol content is below a certain level.

This is called an ignition interlock device, or IID. In the United States, all 50 states have laws requiring people who have been convicted of certain drunk-driving offenses to install an IID in their car for a specific period of time, or at least allowing judges to impose such a requirement. However, you can also *voluntarily* install one in your car; a criminal conviction is not necessary.

If there's an alcoholic in your family, this can be a very good idea. Not only can it prevent alcoholics from being arrested for drunk driving or harming themselves in a crash, but it can also protect your family from devastating legal liability if the alcoholic injures someone else on the road.

Installing such a device might be easier said than done, however. Many alcoholics deeply resent the idea of having such a lock put on their car. Alcoholics who are in denial can be highly insulted by such a clear sign that their family thinks they have a problem. Also, many alcoholics fight the idea because it makes it harder for them to get to a bar or liquor store.

If the car is registered in the alcoholic's name, it can be extremely difficult to install such a device because a voluntary installation usually requires that the registered owner be present or sign an authorization form. In such cases, it might be necessary to make serious threats to get an alcoholic to comply (for example, "I can no longer live with you if you won't take reasonable steps to protect our family by making sure you don't go to jail or lose our home in a lawsuit"). This may be an extreme measure, but it can be warranted if the alcoholic has a history of driving under the influence, and especially if he or she regularly drives with children in the car.

In the United States, the cost of an IID is usually a few dollars per day, plus a fairly modest installation fee.

Alcoholics sometimes try to cheat by getting another person to blow into the tube before they start driving. For this reason, once a car is started, most IID systems will prompt the driver at random intervals to blow into the tube again. Usually the IID will allow the driver sufficient time to pull off the road to do so safely. If the driver fails to blow into the tube or registers a blood alcohol level that is too high, the device will log the incident and initiate some sort of warning, such as turning on the lights and honking the horn repeatedly. The device usually won't shut off the engine, however, because shutting off the engine while the driver is in traffic could be dangerous.

HOME DRUG TESTS

Occasionally families insist that an addict living at home with them submit to regular or random drug tests. For instance, parents of an addicted child might make the tests a condition of being allowed to live at home. Sometimes families ask addicts who are in early recovery to submit to the tests simply so that they can worry less, because during this period many families are obsessive in their anxiety about the possibility of relapse.

Home drug-test kits are available in many pharmacies and online. Some test for one specific drug (such as marijuana, cocaine, or methamphetamines), while others are "multi-panel" and check for a wide variety of substances.

Most home drug tests are urine tests. One problem with these is that a determined addict can sometimes beat them, such as by diluting a urine sample with water, getting a sample from a friend or buying one from someone else, or storing a "clean" sample for use later. Family members can reduce this risk by insisting on watching the addict go to the bathroom, but many family members don't want to do this, and it can make it harder to get the addict to agree to the testing regimen in the first place. (It's also possible to use temperature strips to make sure the urine hasn't been tampered with, but this adds to the cost and complexity.)

Hair follicle tests are also available and generally solve the cheating problem. However, they're usually more expensive and require sending the sample to a lab, so the family has to wait several days for the results.

While most home urine tests are very good, they are never 100 percent accurate. Also, they typically won't pick up very recent drug use, such as use within the last hour or two. With crack cocaine, heroin, and methamphetamines, it can take up to six hours before the drug can be detected in a person's urine, and with ecstasy and benzodiazepines, it can take up to seven hours.

In addition to urine tests for drugs, it's possible to buy portable breath-testing machines for alcohol.

Recently, a new generation of technology has allowed people to blow into a portable device and have their blood alcohol results instantly transmitted to a remote third party for monitoring. These systems are sold with trade names such as Soberlink. The device prompts users to provide a breath sample on a regular basis and then uses cameras or facial recognition technology to make sure the correct person is blowing into the tube.

These systems can be expensive, but they have two big advantages. One is that the alcoholic can be given regular breath tests even when a family member isn't around to administer them. The other is that the alcoholic becomes accountable to a third party, not to a family member. It often creates a lot of interpersonal problems and trust issues when a family member regularly has to take on the role of "cop," and these tensions can be lessened significantly when someone outside the family is doing the monitoring.

With any kind of home drug or alcohol test, a key question that needs to be answered in advance is what will happen if someone tests positive. A positive test can trigger panic, anxiety, and recriminations. Ideally, a family should decide in advance what the consequences will be for a failed test—although in practice this can be difficult to do.

Another question is how often to test. Some families insist on testing a loved one whenever they suspect drug use. This can work, but the problem with testing "on suspicion" is that it can turn every test into a tense drama filled with resentment and responses such as "What did I do to deserve this?" or "Why don't you trust me?" (This is especially true if the addict fears that he or she would fail the test.)

Testing on a regular schedule largely avoids this problem. Of course, it can be difficult to figure out the optimal schedule. Testing too frequently can be a nuisance and can make addicts more likely to object to the program, but testing less frequently can make addicts believe that they can game the system, since they know that after one test is over they won't be tested again for a while.

Some families test randomly. Random testing can be as simple as rolling a pair of dice every night, and if certain numbers come up, a test is required.

HIGH SCHOOL AND COLLEGE PROGRAMS

There are now about 40 high schools in the United States that are designed specifically for students who are in addiction recovery, according to the Association of Recovery Schools, a trade group that supports this type of education.

Recovery schools award a diploma similar to other high schools, but they have special programs to support students in dealing with addiction and co-occurring disorders. Staffing includes both traditional teachers and substance abuse counselors and other mental health professionals.

The schools also typically provide support to families in dealing with addiction and helping young people in recovery.

According to the association, there are eight recovery high schools in California, eight in Texas, six in Minnesota, five in Massachusetts, two in New Jersey, two in Washington state, and one each in Colorado, Florida, Indiana, Oklahoma, Pennsylvania, Rhode Island, Tennessee, Wisconsin, and Wyoming. (New ones may have been opened since this book went to press.)

More specifics are available at the association's website, *www.recoveryschools.org*.

In addition, many colleges and universities now have formal programs for students who are dealing with an addiction, called Collegiate Recovery Programs, or CRPs.

CRPs typically offer on-campus sober housing, Twelve-Step and other self-help meetings, individual counseling, and a recovery-friendly spaces and social environments.

A listing of more than 100 such programs can be found on the website of the Association of Recovery in Higher Education at *www. collegiaterecovery.org*.

WHEN AN ADDICT NEEDS SURGERY

A serious problem can arise if an addict needs to undergo surgery or another treatment that involves a lot of pain. Doctors typically prescribe opioids in connection with such procedures, for anesthesia or for postoperative pain (or both). But this can cause problems for an addict and can make it very difficult for someone in recovery to remain clean and sober. This is true even if the person was addicted to a substance other than opioids because opioids can produce a similar dopamine-related "high."

Of course, the pain of certain medical procedures can be unbearable without drugs. What's more, experiencing tremendous pain after an operation can sometimes keep people from healing as quickly or as well as they otherwise would. As a result, surgery often creates a difficult dilemma.

For people who are in active addiction or very early recovery, one problem is what's called "cross-tolerance." Such patients have usually built up a tolerance to their drug of choice, such that they can take large quantities without experiencing as many effects as other people would. Not only do they have a tolerance to the drug, but they also have a tolerance to other drugs that are chemically similar—a cross-tolerance. As a result, if a doctor prescribes a medication to sedate a patient or put him or her under during a procedure, but the patient turns out to have a cross-tolerance to the drug, the dosage might not work as intended, which can cause serious issues.

For recovering addicts, the most common problem is that being prescribed a lot of opioids in connection with a medical procedure can trigger relapse. But the opposite is also true: If a doctor *underprescribes* pain medication, and the patient experiences a great deal of pain, the patient may seek to self-medicate in an unsupervised way with street drugs, which can start the addiction cycle all over again.

The most important thing in dealing with this issue is to be honest with the medical team about the patient's addiction history. It can also be wise for the medical team to consult with an addiction specialist. There's no perfect solution to the problem, but these two steps can help a great deal.

Some people have tried to manage pain without full-fledged opioids. For example, the drug tramadol is sometimes used with addicts because it is considered to have weaker opioid properties and to be less addictive. Other doctors have attempted to control pain through the use of antidepressants and sleeping pills, although these medications can pose their own risks.

Some people have been able to reduce postsurgical pain through a wearable device that uses electricity to stimulate nerves. This process is called transcutaneous electrical nerve stimulation, or TENS. However, there is conflicting evidence regarding the effectiveness of this method.

Some other high-tech devices designed to reduce pain by disrupting nerve signals to the brain have been approved by the U.S. Food and Drug Administration and are in clinical trials. These devices can be implanted under the skin or worn as patches. They include the Sprint PNS System (for pain in the back and extremities), Stimwave (for chronic pain), Quell (for peripheral pain), and Cefaly (for preventing migraines).

Finally, some people have attempted to reduce pain through meditation and other mindfulness techniques, biofeedback, acupuncture, yoga, and similar methods.

If nothing short of opioids will make a patient's pain bearable, several things can help:

- If possible, it's a good idea for the medication to be dispensed by someone other than the patient, such as a family member. The family member should pick up the medication at the pharmacy and should not keep it on a bedside table or anywhere else that is accessible to the patient.
- Giving pain medication at fixed intervals, rather than "as needed," can be helpful because it doesn't allow the patient to control the drug flow. (It can also reduce conflict between the patient and the person administering the medication.)

- Limiting the duration as much as possible is obviously a good idea.
- Patients should not drink alcohol while taking opioids.
- Family members should dispose of the medication as soon as there is no more need for it. Many pharmacies will take back unused medication for safe disposal.
- Long-acting opioids may be preferable to short-acting ones because the "high" produced by psychotropic drugs is usually related to the speed at which the concentration of the drug increases in the bloodstream.
- Preparing for the period after the operation by planning increased recovery efforts can be a good idea. This can include alerting a sponsor or other members of a support network, scheduling additional therapy sessions, attending more frequent Twelve-Step or other meetings, and arranging for regular drug testing during the months after surgery.

IV

HOW TREATMENT
WORKS

Can Addicts Get Well
without Treatment?

C an you recover from an addiction without any sort of treatment? Sure. You can also have a root canal without Novocain, if you really want to. It's just going to be a whole lot more painful.

Undoubtedly a number of addicts succeed in getting well without treatment. We just have no idea how many there are. The reason is that people don't get officially diagnosed with an addiction unless they're seeing a therapist or otherwise being treated. We can compile statistics about people who seek medical help, but it's impossible to compile statistics about people who *don't* seek medical help.

Many people have heard stories about individuals who used alcohol or drugs excessively and then suddenly stopped, "cold turkey," and never went back. There are even a number of celebrities who fit this category. For instance, President George W. Bush famously quit drinking the day after his 40th birthday party and never used alcohol again. He didn't go to therapy or attend Alcoholics Anonymous, although he did credit his faith for helping him to quit.

Stories like these suggest that a lot of people can recover from an addiction through sheer willpower. The problem, though, is that it's not always clear whether the person in question was really an addict. Remember, addiction isn't defined by how much or how often someone drinks or uses drugs. Addiction is a specific process in the brain, and it's possible to be a very heavy drinker or drug user and not be an addict.

Thus, when we hear these stories, we need to keep in mind that the person who "got over an addiction" through force of will alone might well not really have had an addiction in the first place. (For what it's worth, President Bush said in an interview years later that he had been a very heavy drinker but that he didn't believe he was "clinically an alcoholic. . . . I don't think that was my case.")

It's hard to overestimate the difficulty of getting over a true addiction through sheer willpower, when willpower—the ability of the prefrontal cortex to resist impulses and make reasoned decisions—is exactly what the disease targets and dismantles. That's not to say that it can't be done, but it's extraordinarily difficult.

Quite a few addicts insist to their loved ones that they don't need treatment and that they can get over their problem by themselves. Most often this is a form of denial. Either because of defensiveness or because the prefrontal cortex isn't working properly, addicts often don't truly understand that they have a problem, and so they don't think they need help to fix it.

In Alcoholics Anonymous, people who try to give up alcohol without any sort of treatment are often said to be "white-knuckling it." The image is of someone holding on for dear life, like a very frightened person on a roller coaster.

In theory, if such people held on long enough, they could get through the withdrawal symptoms and the cravings. Their brains would slowly start to heal, and they could once again lead a normal life. In reality, though, a very large number of "white-knucklers" can't hold out, and relapse.

The goal of treatment is to slow down the roller coaster and make it easier to hang on. Treatment helps addicts understand how they got into the situation they're in and gives them helpful coping mechanisms for avoiding relapse temptations and handling difficult life situations. It can include drugs to make withdrawal easier and reduce cravings. And it can include support groups that allow addicts to talk through their problems and get reinforcement for making better choices.

Another common AA term for a person who is trying to stop drinking without treatment is a "dry drunk." The implication is that such people may be managing to avoid alcohol for now, but they haven't turned their life around in other ways and built a new, constructive lifestyle based on something other than substances. In other words, they are practicing abstinence but are not truly in recovery.

None of this is to say that a person can't get well without treatment. But experience tends to show that the vast majority of people can't, or at least that they can't for a sustained period of time.

One final note: It can be dangerous to try to stop using two particular substances—alcohol and benzodiazepines—cold turkey on your own because sudden withdrawal can cause a risk of seizures. It's especially important for people who have been abusing these substances and want to quit to do so in a medically controlled way.

22

A Brief Overview
of Treatment Options

One of the things that makes addiction such a difficult problem is that there is no one treatment protocol that works for everyone. Different types of treatment work better for different people, and there's often no good way to tell in advance which approaches are likely to be the most successful for a given individual. For this reason, it can be a good idea to try a number of different types of treatment to see which ones work best.

The problem is compounded because, in the United States and many other countries, there's ordinarily no one doctor or other professional who will take charge of the problem and arrange for various types of treatment. Figuring out what to do is usually left up to the addict—or, in a great many cases, the family.

It's odd that this is so. More and more people refer to addiction as a disease, but it's often not treated as a disease by the medical system. If you develop a "normal" disease such as diabetes or cancer, you typically have a specialized professional put in charge of your care who decides what types of treatment are appropriate for you and makes sure you receive them. It isn't left up to the patient's family to figure out whether the patient should receive cancer surgery or radiation or chemotherapy, for instance—and the family doesn't have to search the Internet or perform other types of research to figure out who is a qualified treatment provider. Yet with addiction, it's very often the patient's family members who have to educate themselves about the problem and decide on the best course of action.

It's not clear why this is the case. It may partly be the legacy of many years of addiction being thought of as a bad moral choice rather than a disease or a psychological disorder. But it might also be due to the fact that addiction treatment falls into many different realms— medicine, pharmacology, psychiatry, social work, and self-help groups run by and for addicts. Very few professionals are competent to act as experts in all these fields.

The practical result, though, is that it's common for no one outside the family to be in charge and for treatment to be provided in a piece-meal manner. For instance, a hospital emergency room might handle the immediate symptoms of a heroin overdose or alcohol poisoning, but it will often discharge the patient without any significant effort to address the underlying problem that caused the hospital visit in the first place.

This is incredibly difficult for family members. The family is already overburdened just trying to cope with the addict's behavior, yet on top of this they're expected to do research and make treatment decisions that would be challenging even for highly skilled professionals.

FIVE TYPES OF TREATMENT

Five basic types of treatment are used for addicts, all of which are dis-cussed in more detail in the following chapters:

Detoxification, or **detox,** is an acute inpatient (and sometimes out-patient) program. Detox is for weaning addicts off their substance of choice in a safe manner, and is not meant as a long-term method of helping addicts recover. The goal is simply to get them off alcohol or drugs right now, to prevent harm while doing so, and to make them better able to take advantage of other, longer-term types of treatment.

Rehabilitation, or **rehab,** is a controlled setting where addicts who have been through detox (or abstained for a requisite period) can go for intensive treatments, usually consisting of some combination of the three methods that follow. Rehab offers a structured environment where addicts can begin the healing process away from the temptation of drugs, alcohol, gambling opportunities, and so forth. It typically lasts anywhere from a week to several months and can involve a full-time residential facility or a part-time day program.

Psychotherapy is used to help addicts understand their own minds more fully, so they can make better choices and resist temptations. A wide variety of psychotherapeutic approaches are available. Some are designed to address underlying emotional issues that may have caused the addict to start using in the first place. Some are more present-oriented and try to equip addicts with practical tools to help them recognize what triggers cravings, avoid dangerous situations, and make good decisions.

Drug treatments are designed to help addicts resist cravings and improve their emotional outlook. These treatments take a number of different approaches and can vary depending on the addict's substance of choice.

Support groups allow addicts to meet and address their concerns in a mutually supportive environment. The most common type of support group is a Twelve-Step program, although there are others. These groups are typically not administered by a doctor or treatment facility, but instead are run by recovering addicts themselves.

In addition to these more formal treatments, many recovering addicts make an effort to adopt healthier lifestyle habits. These can include exercise programs, yoga, and mindfulness techniques such as meditation. These are not treatment methods *per se*, but they often accompany treatment programs and can be very helpful to people who are making a major change in their life.

• • • • • • • **23** • • • • • • •

What Really Happens
in Detox?

The goal of detox is to wean addicts off whatever substances they're using and to do so in a medically safe manner. Detox is not a full-fledged form of addiction treatment in itself, and it's different from rehab (although detox and rehab are often confused, especially by tabloid newspapers reporting on troubled starlets). Detox is simply a first step—it's a way to get addicts clean and sober so they can *then* undergo long-term treatment.

Detox programs can operate on either an inpatient or an outpatient basis. Outpatient detox—where the addict is allowed to go home at night—*can* work, but its track record is not as good. Outpatient detox has the best chance of success if an addiction is not very severe, if the addict is highly motivated to seek help, and if there is considerable family support. In many cases, though, the temptation to relapse at night is simply too great. For this reason, inpatient detox is the more reliable option.

An inpatient detox facility is usually a locked ward, where access from the outside is strictly limited and patients are allowed outdoors only under highly supervised conditions. This is necessary to make sure that addicts have no access to contraband while undergoing withdrawal. Such facilities also typically ban additional items such as electronics and prescription medications (which may be confiscated and then administered by a doctor).

Detox usually starts with an intake process, which can involve a lot of paperwork. Once the addict is admitted, medical personnel will take a drug history and perform a medical exam and a psychological assessment to create a personalized treatment plan. The addict's belongings will also be searched for contraband.

The length of detox depends a great deal on the substances the addict was using, the severity of the addiction, and the addict's general physical health. Detox generally lasts from a few days to a few weeks, but a stay of under a week is not uncommon.

As the substances leave the addict's system, some symptoms of withdrawal are likely to occur. These can range from mood swings, anxiety, and irritability to headaches and muscle aches, nausea, vomiting, depression, panic attacks, insomnia, trembling and shaking, fever, and even hallucinations in some cases. Medicine is often given to the addict to reduce cravings and alleviate withdrawal symptoms. Doctors will usually monitor addicts carefully, at least once a day, to help them cope and to assess their progress.

Although the goal of detox is to wean the addict off substances, not to provide long-term care, it's not uncommon for detox facilities to provide some sort of additional treatment during the addict's stay. Most commonly, this includes support group–style meetings and discussions. Psychotherapy is less common, given the temporary nature of detox, but doctors may prescribe some of the same sorts of medications that would be used in long-term drug therapy.

When choosing a detox facility, some good questions to ask are:

- Is it accredited by the Joint Commission (the national organization that accredits health care facilities) and licensed by the state licensing authority?
- Does it regularly treat the addict's substance of choice?
- Is a medical doctor on staff or on call 24 hours a day?
- Are the other treatment professionals licensed or credentialed?
- What is the patient-to-staff ratio?
- What insurance is accepted?
- Does it provide access to Twelve-Step or other support-group meetings?
- Does it offer individualized treatment plans?
- How helpful is it in referring patients to rehabs or otherwise developing an aftercare plan?

THE DANGER OF "SELF-DETOX"

Addicts, especially if they become desperate and don't have strong support systems, sometimes try to "self-detox" by simply giving up a substance and going cold turkey. This can actually be medically dangerous, especially with certain substances.

One thing that surprises many people is that you're actually more at risk for death if you suddenly stop drinking alcohol than if you suddenly stop taking heroin. The agony of heroin withdrawal is well known in certain parts of popular culture, but heroin withdrawal by itself is virtually never fatal (unless the addict has other complicating factors). However, a person who suddenly withdraws from excessive alcohol consumption could experience a seizure, which could be deadly.

There have been cases where a family member is taking an alcoholic to a detox facility and the facility instructs the family member to stop at a liquor store along the way and make the alcoholic take a drink. This typically comes as quite a shock to the family member, but it could potentially be life-saving advice if the person has recently been drinking heavily and has suddenly stopped.

Other dangerous drugs from which to withdraw are benzodiazepines, which have a similar seizure risk.

While heroin withdrawal isn't fatal in and of itself, it can put addicts in a more dangerous position if they relapse. Withdrawal changes the addict's level of tolerance, so that if the addict then goes out and uses the same dose that he or she did before, there's a much greater risk of overdose.

It's not uncommon to hear tragic stories of heroin addicts who finally made it to detox, only to die of an overdose shortly afterward. What most people who hear these stories don't realize is the likely causal connection between the two.

• • • • • • • **24** • • • • • • •

What Really Happens
in Rehab?

Rehabilitation, or rehab, is a broad term that encompasses a wide variety of programs designed to treat addiction and promote recovery. Rehabs can range from a bare-bones outpatient program that addicts attend for a few hours a day to a luxurious spa-like setting where addicts can spend several months, at a cost well into six figures.

Rehab is *not* a kind of treatment in and of itself. Rather, it's a controlled environment where an addict can avoid the temptation of using substances while taking advantage of educational programs and some or all of the three main kinds of actual treatment—psychotherapy, drug treatments, and support groups. In this sense, a rehab facility is like a hospital—no one gets better simply by walking into a hospital; it's just a location where various health services can be provided in an intensive setting.

Rehab programs are not centrally regulated, and there is no one single general principle for how they operate. Different programs can have very different approaches and emphases, which is why it's wise to research them carefully before signing up.

Is rehab necessary? That depends. Rehab isn't necessary in the sense that many people have recovered from addiction without it, usually by engaging on their own in one or more of the three main treatment methods listed earlier. However, a good rehab program can provide addicts with a leg up in recovery by focusing their efforts, connecting them with resources, and giving them a space where they can avoid the distractions and temptations of everyday life.

In addition to the three main forms of treatment, rehabs sometimes provide other types of help to addicts. Many offer classes geared to developing healthy lifestyle habits. Some (although by no means all) offer assistance with housing, employment, education, financial problems, and legal issues.

WHERE REHAB CAME FROM

Rehab began as a social reform movement in the United States in the 1950s. At the time, alcoholics and drug addicts were frequently locked up in mental hospitals, and the conditions were often abysmal. Several reformers came up with a new concept, in which addicts could live together in a kind of rooming house. There were house rules, and sobriety was enforced, but addicts were treated with dignity. Treatment consisted almost entirely of the Twelve-Step model, and there was an emphasis on providing education to addicts and their families.

A key early adopter of this approach was the Hazelden Foundation in Minnesota, and the approach came to be called the "Minnesota Model." Most rehab programs today derive in some fairly direct way from the Minnesota Model. Perhaps for this reason, the vast majority of rehabs in the United States rely to a large degree on the Twelve Steps.

(By the way, the country's most famous rehab, the Betty Ford Center, merged with the Hazelden Foundation in 2014. It's now called the Hazelden Betty Ford Foundation.)

Another influential component of the Minnesota Model was the idea of treatment being provided by a combination of trained medical staff and recovering addicts. Today many rehabs employ a significant number of addicts in recovery to provide help to patients.

This has benefits and drawbacks. Recovering addicts can sometimes communicate especially well with patients because they can relate to their experience in a very direct way. Patients often find them credible and helpful. On the other hand, in practice many such employees are hired with very little in the way of experience, education, or professional credentials other than their background as addicts. This creates some potential for making mistakes, especially with patients who suffer from other complex psychological disorders in addition to addiction.

INPATIENT OR OUTPATIENT?

While people often speak of "going away to rehab," residential programs are in fact less common than partial-day programs. The majority of people who sign up for rehab attend an outpatient program. (And this has become especially true lately in the United States as insurance companies have cut back on their coverage of residential programs.)

There's no one right answer for everyone as to whether an inpatient or outpatient program is best. A number of studies have attempted to compare treatment outcomes (i.e., how long people are able to stay clean and sober) between the two. The results are mixed. Some studies show that outpatient facilities are just as good as residential programs—and these studies are often happily cited by the insurance industry. However, these studies may be of limited value because other research has shown that the people who go to outpatient programs tend to be a very different population from those who go to residential programs. For example, they tend to be better educated, more likely to be employed, less severe in their usage, less likely to have had other treatment before that was unsuccessful, and less likely to suffer from other mental health problems.

This means that, in general, addicts who go to outpatient programs tend to be less sick and have a better prognosis than addicts in residential programs. So while studies may show that outpatient programs have results that are just as good as inpatient programs, that doesn't actually mean that the treatment is just as effective. The studies are comparing apples and oranges.

Obviously, inpatient programs are more expensive and preclude someone from returning to work or family responsibilities. Much depends on the family's financial situation and the addict's individual needs.

Inpatient rehab might be a better idea for people—especially young adults—who would otherwise go right back to the same friends and environments where they were used to using drugs. It might also be better for people who need treatment for co-occurring disorders, people for whom the chances of relapse are particularly high, and people who want or need to develop healthier lifestyle habits. (It's more common for higher-end inpatient rehabs to offer amenities such as personal training and fitness, yoga, meditation, and art therapy.)

Some people plan to start off at an outpatient rehab and switch to an inpatient rehab later if they find that they need more support. (In fact, some insurance companies require addicts to try an outpatient program first before they will cover an inpatient program; see Chapter 25.)

On the other hand, many people start off with a stint at a residential facility and then "step down" to a day program.

Some outpatient programs specialize in particular professions—police and firefighters, for example. For addicts who belong to such a group, entering a program with their peers can be very helpful.

WHAT'S A TYPICAL DAY LIKE?

While some residential rehabs appear from the outside like resorts, almost all of them have fairly strict controls. Visits from family and friends are limited and regulated. Mail and packages are subject to search. Patients may go "off-site" only at certain times and generally only under a counselor's supervision. The daily schedule is highly regimented, including wake-up and bedtimes, and "free time" occurs only in scheduled blocks. Attendance at therapy sessions and meetings is mandatory.

Following is a typical daily schedule from the Fernside program operated by McLean Hospital in Massachusetts. It's reprinted here because it's fairly representative of daily schedules in inpatient rehab programs:

8:30 A.M.: Goals group

9:00 A.M.: Group meetings (depending on the day, acceptance and commitment therapy, emotion regulation, self-esteem, mindfulness, or men's and women's groups)

10:00 A.M.: Psychology education

11:00 A.M.: Individual meetings

12:00 P.M.: Lunch

1:00 P.M.: Group meetings (depending on the day, cognitive-behavioral therapy, interpersonal effectiveness training, distress tolerance, or group therapy)

2:00 P.M.: Narrative groups

3:00 P.M.: Fitness, yoga, or expressive therapy

5:00 P.M.: Skills practice

5:30 P.M.: Dinner

7:00 P.M.: Twelve-Step or other self-help meetings

10:00 P.M.: Wrap-up

As for outpatient programs, the daily schedule is generally similar but more compressed. Also, outpatient programs typically start each day with a drug or alcohol test to make sure the patient hasn't relapsed overnight.

HOW LONG SHOULD AN ADDICT STAY?

There is no ideal length of stay in rehab, despite the prevalent idea in popular culture that a "standard" stay is 28 days. (Indeed, in 2000 there was a Hollywood movie about rehab that was called *28 Days*.)

As with many things in rehab, the 28-day concept is a product of the Minnesota Model. Early on in the Minnesota programs, there was a general "rule of thumb" that it took about four weeks for alcoholics to get the alcohol out of their system, adapt to the rehab surroundings and routine, and become generally stabilized. When insurance companies later began covering substance abuse treatment, they turned to this "rule of thumb," and many policies were written so as to cover rehab programs for 28 days. This led to the popular idea that 28 days is the norm.

But there is nothing magical about 28 days. Every addict is different, and every addict has different needs. Plus, while the 28-day rule of thumb was derived from early experience with alcoholics, many insurance companies now apply it to rehab for other substances, such as opioids, where it might be even less appropriate. (While everyone is different, many experts believe that opioid addicts in general tend to need longer treatment than alcoholics.)

Some rehab programs require a minimum stay of 30 days, believing that anything less than that won't give an addict a reasonable chance at recovery. And many experts now believe that addicts still tend to be "shaky" and excessively prone to relapse even after 30 days and that 90 days in a controlled environment is necessary for ideal treatment.

Of course, to the extent that rehab works, anything is better than nothing. Some addicts attend an outpatient program for only a week and find it very helpful.

• • • • • • • 25 • • • • • • •

How to Find a Good Rehab—
and Pay for It

U nfortunately, there is no truly reliable directory of top-quality
rehab programs. Some rehabs advertise heavily online and have
beautiful websites, but all that tells you is that a particular rehab facility
has a large public relations budget, not that it's a good value or that it
provides excellent care. And many online directories of rehabs don't list
all of them, just the ones that pay to be in the directory.

Often the best way to find a good rehab is to get a referral from
someone you trust who can recommend something based on your particular needs. Many good detox facilities can recommend an appropriate
rehab as part of their aftercare planning. Doctors and therapists who
specialize in addiction can also be a good resource.

WHAT TO ASK

In researching rehabs, a good first question is whether the facility is
accredited. The two main accrediting organizations are the Commission on Accreditation of Rehabilitation Facilities, or CARF, and the
Joint Commission. (The Joint Commission was formerly called the
Joint Commission on Accreditation of Healthcare Organizations and is
still occasionally referred to as JCAHO or "jay-co.")

You may want to ask how many doctors, psychologists, and licensed social workers are on staff. Be careful—in some facilities these professionals are truly on staff; in others they are associated with the facility but just occasionally drop in.

Other good questions include whether there will be a single case manager to oversee all of the addict's care and what role the facility will expect the family to play in treatment.

If the addict has another mental health disorder in addition to the addiction, you'll want to know what specialized treatment options are offered.

Some rehabs are highly focused on Twelve-Step programs, while others offer a variety of treatments including behavioral therapy. You'll want to know about the facility's treatment philosophy, particularly if you have doubts about whether a Twelve-Step program will work in your case.

If a facility offers cognitive-behavioral therapy or motivational interviewing, and these approaches are important to you, it's a good idea to find out what training or certification the providers have. (See Chapter 26 for more information on these types of therapies.) Many rehabs claim to offer cognitive-behavioral therapy or motivational interviewing, but the providers aren't properly trained or the methods they use deviate from what's generally accepted by experts. In some cases, this can amount to a kind of false advertising.

If the addict is a teenager, you might want to consider rehabs that specialize in teenagers. This is often a better idea than a rehab that lumps teenagers and adults together because teenagers often have special needs and tend to fare better when they are surrounded by their peers. (Adults might also want to inquire if the facility includes teenagers because they might feel that they would do better in an environment consisting only of *their* peers.)

Some rehabs that focus on teenagers are "wilderness" programs that offer treatment in a camp-style environment with similarities to an Outward Bound program. A few follow a "boot camp" model, with a military-style environment and a strict regimen including exercise and chores.

Proximity is another issue. A nearby rehab will mean fewer travel costs and more chances for family to visit. But sometimes spending time away from a familiar environment can help an addict make a clean break and start over fresh.

A potentially useful book that contains numerous descriptive stories about experiences in different types of rehabs is *Inside Rehab* by Anne M. Fletcher.

PAYING FOR REHAB

In the United States and some other countries, often the most difficult thing about rehab is paying for it. Some form of rehab is frequently covered by private health insurance, but rehab can be expensive, and limits may apply.

Parity

In 2008, the U.S. Congress passed a law saying that if a group health insurance plan—the kind offered by most employers—offers benefits for both (1) medical and surgical expenses and (2) mental health and substance abuse expenses, it has to offer "parity" between the two. That means that mental health and substance abuse expenses must be covered at least as generously in terms of copays, deductibles, limits on the number of visits or days of coverage, and so forth.

This law has generally made it easier for addicts and their families to get insurance coverage for rehab programs. On the other hand, the law applies only to group plans, and it doesn't say that these plans *have* to cover addiction and other mental health problems—only that if they do, they must offer parity.

In 2010, the Affordable Care Act extended the requirements of the 2008 law to *individual* health care policies as well, with limited exceptions. And in 2014, the Affordable Care Act began requiring that individual health plans that are offered on the marketplace exchange cover substance abuse treatment and offer parity.

A useful website that explains how the U.S. parity laws apply to your specific situation, run by the U.S. Department of Health and Human Services, is *www.hhs.gov/programs/topic-sites/mental-health-parity/mental-health-and-addiction-insurance-help/index.html.*

Qualifying for Insurance

If rehab is covered by an insurance policy, you'll want to check the policy to see what it covers and also contact the insurance company for clarification once you have a particular treatment plan in mind. Be persistent—many people who were initially denied coverage have nevertheless succeeded by calling back repeatedly and asking to speak to higher-level managers.

The rehab facility itself may be willing to contact your insurance company and negotiate on your behalf. Often a facility has a great deal of experience in working with insurers, and it will have an incentive to get you covered.

Some insurance policies may require an addict to complete an outpatient treatment program before applying for benefits for inpatient treatment. Also, if an addict has another mental health disorder in addition to the addiction, you'll want to ask how this will be handled. Some companies treat co-occurring disorders as a single illness, and some break them out as two different illnesses. This can affect the timing of when you reach the maximum coverage.

In the United States, both Medicare and Medicaid generally cover addiction treatment.

Other Ways to Cover the Cost

If you have trouble getting insurance coverage for rehab, here are some other ideas:

- Many businesses offer employee assistance programs, or EAPs, and these sometimes help with rehab costs.
- The U.S. Department of Veterans Affairs offers some rehab services at VA hospitals.
- Most U.S. states (and even a few cities) offer rehab grants for people who can't afford treatment. Contacting a department of health or human services may help. (There are often waiting lists for these programs, however.)
- The Salvation Army offers free rehab programs for people who can't afford treatment. Most of these are in the United States, but there are programs in Canada, the United Kingdom, Australia,

New Zealand, and a number of other countries. To participate, you must be willing to work 40 hours a week for the organization (usually at a Salvation Army store) and be willing to participate in Christian meetings and Bible study in addition to Twelve-Step meetings.

- Some people can ask for help (as a loan or a gift) from relatives. Generally, the relative will insist on paying the rehab directly rather than giving cash to the addict, to make sure that the money won't be spent on drugs instead. Affluent families that make large gifts or loans for this purpose should contact a tax advisor because tax issues may arise.

Paying for rehab can be an even bigger problem if an addict relapses, and it can become extraordinarily difficult if an addict relapses multiple times. While insurance might cover part of the cost of a first stint in rehab, getting coverage for a subsequent stay can be very difficult.

• • • • • • • **26** • • • • • • • •

Psychotherapy Approaches That Are Used for Addicts

The goal of psychotherapy is to help people better understand what's going on when they're tempted to engage in self-destructive behaviors, so they can stop engaging in them. The premise is that *the mind can heal itself*—when people are more aware of what they're doing, they have more control over whether to do it.

This is important for addiction, since the central problem for addicts is that their free will is impaired and they can't make voluntary choices. The aim of therapy is to lift the veil so that the addict can see what's happening and regain a measure of free will.

There are two basic schools of thought when it comes to psychotherapy for addicts.

On the one hand, traditional psychotherapy focuses on *why* addicts behave as they do. It looks for reasons or experiences in their history that might explain what causes them to rely on a substance. In this sense, traditional psychotherapy is *past-focused.*

In contrast, there is a wide variety of newer behavioral approaches and therapies. These therapies are not particularly interested in the *why* of the addict's behavior or what might have happened long ago in the person's childhood. Rather, they try to understand what behaviors need to be modified right now, how the addict is thinking in the present that leads to these behaviors, and what changes in attitudes or reasoning might be made to reduce them. These approaches are more interested in the *what* of the addict's behavior and are more *present-focused.*

The two approaches are not mutually exclusive. Indeed, some addicts in rehab are exposed to both kinds of therapy, more or less with the attitude of "Hey, whatever works!" However, it's important to note that most therapists are trained in one school of thought and will probably be able to apply only one of the approaches. For this reason, it's important to know which approach a therapist will use and to be comfortable with it. (Some therapists who prefer one approach can actually be quite antagonistic or dismissive toward the other one.)

TRADITIONAL PSYCHOTHERAPY

Traditional psychotherapy (often referred to as "talk therapy") traces its roots back to Sigmund Freud, although the practice has changed a great deal since nineteenth-century Vienna.

Freud pioneered the idea that our minds don't always know themselves completely. He believed that certain thoughts, desires, and experiences are too painful or embarrassing for us to experience consciously and, as a result, we repress them. They don't disappear, however; rather, the repressed thoughts go into a part of our mind called the unconscious.

But putting a thought, desire, or experience into the unconscious isn't like storing it in the attic and forgetting about it. The thought is still present, and it wants to get out. Because it can't get out consciously, it expresses itself in some other way.

In some cases, this expression can be relatively harmless. For instance, Freud thought that many slips of the tongue were actually the result of unconscious thoughts bubbling up to the surface. (Hence the phrase "Freudian slip.")

But other times, unconscious thoughts can manifest themselves in destructive behaviors, such as neuroses. Freud came up with psychoanalysis as a "talking cure" in which a troubled patient, guided by a therapist, reflects on the behavior and gradually comes to understand the underlying unconscious impulse behind it. Freud believed that once the unconscious cause of the behavior was brought into the light of day, and the patient understood the *why* of the behavior, he or she could freely choose to stop engaging in it.

Much has changed in psychotherapy, and there are very few strict Freudians today, but these basic concepts still undergird a great deal of the traditional psychotherapeutic approach.

The application to addiction is fairly clear: Addicts, like neurotics, lack free will with regard to their behavior. Something is causing them to behave in a destructive way, and they don't know what it is, nor can they consciously control it. So, traditional psychotherapy delves into the addict's past and tries to understand what hidden impulses, hurts, or trauma are behind the addictive "acting out." The idea is that, if the addict finally comes to terms with the underlying issue and makes it conscious, he or she can then *consciously* choose whether to continue drinking or using drugs.

To take an example: Suppose an addict had a traumatic experience in the past that caused him to feel helpless, anxious, or out of control. Perhaps he had a domineering father, or he was bullied, or he was in an abusive relationship, or any of hundreds of other explanations. Because the experience was painful, he repressed it. However, whenever he feels a little bit helpless or anxious in the present day due to the normal ebb and flow of life, this experience is greatly magnified for him because it triggers unconscious associations with the earlier trauma. As a result, he drinks to self-medicate against the flood of anxiety. He literally doesn't know why he needs to drink because the actual root cause remains unconscious. Through therapy, however, he may uncover his earlier, repressed feelings. Once these feelings become conscious, he can deal with them properly, and the need to drink to cope with them will be greatly reduced.

Does It Work?

Does this approach work? As with most treatments in the area of addiction, it works *for some people*. A number of addicts have been helped greatly by it.

Of course, as with most addiction treatments, there are also some negatives. One is that this type of treatment takes time. It can take many months or years of talking and self-reflection to uncover one's unconscious impulses. Many people need more immediate forms of treatment in addition to using therapy as a long-term solution. And many people cannot afford to pay for a treatment that lasts so long.

A second issue with traditional psychotherapy has to do with Freud's idea that once the unconscious is made conscious, free will is restored and the patient can make a reasoned decision. With addiction, however, the brain has been hijacked by a substance and has changed at a chemical level. A breakthrough on a psychiatrist's couch may be wonderful, but it doesn't do anything to adjust the patient's dopamine level or the number of dopamine receptors in the brain, which means that there are still strong physiological headwinds that may prevent the person from making truly voluntary choices.

This is another reason traditional psychotherapy may best be viewed as a long-term aid in managing addiction as a chronic disease, as opposed to a short-term solution for someone in crisis.

BEHAVIORAL THERAPIES

Behavioral therapies are much less interested in the unconscious or in what past event might be triggering present-day destructive tendencies. These newer approaches are based on the idea that the addict is simply *thinking poorly about the issue.* The addict is making incorrect assumptions, using faulty reasoning, or responding inappropriately to stimuli, which results in maladaptive behavior. The goal of these therapies is to identify addicts' mental mistakes and to equip them with better ways of thinking and better coping strategies so they can make better decisions.

Unlike traditional psychotherapy, which treats the symptoms of a psychological illness as reflecting some much deeper problem, behavioral approaches tend to assume that *the symptoms are the problem.* Attack and eliminate the symptoms and you eliminate the problem.

Many of these therapies are referred to as "evidence-based," because you can produce evidence as to whether they work. For instance, if the goal is to reduce drinking, and the average patient is drinking 40 percent less after six months of treatment, that's hard evidence of success. (By contrast, you can't quantify a psychological insight into the unconscious.)

Another difference is that behavioral therapies tend to view the psychologist–patient relationship as more collegial, as a pair working together as a team to solve a problem, in contrast to traditional psychotherapy where the therapist acts more as a guide.

There are a large number of behavioral therapies, but the following are the most common ones used in the treatment of addiction.

Cognitive-Behavioral Therapy

Cognitive-behavioral therapy, or CBT, is the result of a merger of two older types of treatment, which were called (not surprisingly) cognitive therapy and behavioral therapy.

Cognitive therapy was developed by a psychiatrist named Aaron Beck. Beck believed that many psychological problems were caused not by negative experiences being repressed into the unconscious but by people simply drawing the wrong conclusions from such experiences. People made mental errors and began thinking in inappropriately negative ways. Beck believed that he could solve problems simply by changing the way people interpreted events and fit them into the larger picture of their lives—in other words, by changing their cognition.

As for behavioral therapy, it was based on studies of how people are conditioned to respond in certain ways to certain stimuli and how they can be retrained in more positive ways. One of the leading pioneers in this field was Ivan Pavlov, who was famous for showing that if a dog was fed every time it heard the sound of a metronome, eventually it would start to salivate whenever it heard the sound, even if no food was present.

CBT starts by identifying problematic behaviors and establishing a baseline, so that how often the behaviors occur can be shown clearly. The goal is then to measurably reduce the frequency of the behaviors. This is done by focusing on the thoughts and feelings that accompany the behaviors and trying to get the patient to reconsider whether those thoughts and feelings are in fact valid.

To take an example: A woman loses her job and begins feeling incompetent and worthless. As a result of these feelings, she avoids seeking another job for fear of being further exposed as incompetent. Or she may seek another job but be unsuccessful because she gives off a "vibe" of worthlessness. Her inability to find work then reinforces her sense of incompetence, which produces a vicious circle. And of course, her unhappiness and lack of self-esteem may trigger drinking or drug use.

CBT targets the "I'm worthless" thought pattern and challenges it. The goal is to get the woman to consider other possibilities—perhaps she was a bad fit for the old job, or perhaps her boss just didn't understand the value of her contribution. The therapist might also get her to engage in more positive actions, such as considering what job would be a better fit and taking steps to look for work.

Finally, the therapy seeks to give the woman mental skills so that when negative thoughts arise, she can recognize them as such and challenge them with a more positive interpretation of events. In a sense, CBT seeks to empower the patient to become her own therapist.

In the case of addiction, CBT tries to understand the thoughts and ideas that specifically lead to substance abuse and to replace them with more positive interpretations and choices.

CBT requires a good deal of specialized training. Some rehabs and other institutions claim to offer CBT, but in fact the providers aren't properly trained or don't follow accepted practices. If you're interested in this approach, it's a good idea to inquire about the provider's background and training.

In the United States, the National Association of Cognitive-Behavioral Therapists certifies providers. A Certified Cognitive-Behavioral Group Facilitator (CBGF) has completed a home-study program. A Certified Cognitive-Behavioral Group Therapist (CBGT) also has a master's degree in mental health. A Certified Cognitive-Behavioral Therapist (CCBT) has a master's degree and six years of experience and has completed specialized coursework. A Diplomate in Cognitive-Behavioral Therapy (DCBT) must meet all these requirements plus have 10 years of experience, meet continuing education requirements, and publish at least one relevant article each year.

It's possible to be a good CBT practitioner without certification, but certification assures you that the therapist has received at least some relevant training.

Motivational Interviewing

Motivational interviewing, or MI, is designed to help people make changes in their life (such as stopping substance abuse) by focusing intensely on their motivation for change.

MI assumes that people who are struggling with change are experiencing some ambivalence or conflicting feelings. The goal of MI is to identify, examine, and resolve these feelings. The therapist asks a lot of questions to help the person understand his or her conflicting motivations and work through them to a decision.

A key principle of MI is that the therapist is a collaborator, and the goal is for people to come to their own decisions, not simply to reach a decision favored by the therapist.

As with CBT, a number of rehabs and other institutions claim to offer MI, but not everyone who provides it has the proper training and background.

Motivational Enhancement Therapy

Closely related to MI is motivational enhancement therapy, or MET. The two use similar methods, but MET usually begins with a detailed assessment of the person's current drug usage and then provides feedback about changes in that usage. Also, whereas MI involves a broad examination of the person's attitude toward substances, MET tends to focus more specifically on ambivalent feelings about going into a treatment program.

Research suggests that MET is more effective with alcohol and marijuana than with heroin or cocaine.

Both MI and MET are typically short-term therapies, often lasting about four sessions. The goal is not to provide long-term support but to help people decide for themselves about engaging in other practices that will help change their behavior.

Dialectical Behavior Therapy

Dialectical behavior therapy, or DBT, is an offshoot of CBT that was developed in the 1970s by psychologist Marsha Linehan. Linehan believed that certain people are prone to have much more emotional responses than others in interpersonal situations, particularly those involving family, friends, and romantic partners. As you can imagine, these people are especially likely to get into negative thought loops of the kind that CBT tries to remedy.

The main goal of DBT is to help people cope with difficult emotional and interpersonal situations without resorting to self-destructive behaviors (such as drinking or using drugs). Of course, DBT can be helpful for anyone who has an addiction problem, not just people who are especially emotional.

Mindfulness exercises play a key role in DBT. Many of these are derived from Buddhist meditative practices, although DBT adapts them without any religious content. The goal of DBT mindfulness is to develop the ability to be cognizant of the present situation without attaching an emotional reaction to it—to be fully in the moment and aware but nonjudgmental.

Closely related to mindfulness is "distress tolerance"—exercises where one learns to apply the same nonjudgmental, observational attitude in situations that may be particularly emotionally upsetting.

"Emotion regulation" exercises teach people how to identify and label their emotions and be more aware of their emotional reactions, so they can choose not to respond emotionally to certain situations or to apply more positive emotions.

Finally, "interpersonal effectiveness" exercises are similar to assertiveness-training classes. They teach people how to ask for what they want, say no, and cope effectively with interpersonal conflict.

Acceptance and Commitment Therapy

Acceptance and commitment therapy, or ACT, takes the mindfulness approach of DBT to an extreme. It believes that people should not struggle against unpleasant experiences or negative thought loops, but simply be mindfully aware of them and not overreact to them.

ACT tends to reject any attempt to formulate behaviors as "psychological problems" or "symptoms," believing that calling something a problem only makes it harder to let go of it. ACT encourages people to accept negative thoughts and experiences for what they are and to commit to more positive responses.

There are few if any statistical studies proving that DBT and ACT are effective with addiction. However, the techniques are often used for addicts, particularly those who also have a separate mental health issue.

Twelve-Step Facilitation

Twelve-Step facilitation, or TSF, is a therapy designed to support and encourage participation in a Twelve-Step support group such as Alcoholics Anonymous. (Twelve-Step programs are discussed in Chapters 29 and 30.)

TSF sessions usually last about 12 weeks, unlike Twelve-Step programs, where members are encouraged to participate indefinitely.

Also, unlike Twelve-Step groups themselves, TSF is usually thought of as an evidence-based behavioral technique.

Family Behavior Therapy

Family behavior therapy, or FBT, usually lasts about six months and involves therapy sessions with an addict and at least one family member. It's based on the Community Reinforcement Approach (discussed in Chapter 12) of reducing substance dependence by adjusting the person's environment. There's a lot of emphasis on developing skills to avoid drug-related situations, develop social relationships with people who don't use drugs, find a job or do better at work or in school, and relate better within the family.

FBT often involves making a contract with rewards and consequences for different behaviors.

DO BEHAVIORAL THERAPIES WORK?

As with traditional psychotherapy, behavioral therapies work for some people. Their main advantages are that they are quicker and more directly focused on immediate results. Studies tend to show that behavioral therapies work better than talk therapy at getting people in active addiction stabilized and helping them to achieve abstinence. They can also be particularly effective for addicts in early recovery, who are often fragile and in need of practical coping skills to deal with stressful situations and avoid relapse.

Of course, one problem with behavioral therapies is the same as with traditional psychotherapy—they don't address the chemical changes in the brain. It's hard enough to alter negative thought patterns or overcome ambivalence in general, but it's even more difficult when the brain's own reward system is sending powerful contradictory messages. For this reason, both types of therapies are often used in conjunction with drug treatments, which can mitigate some of the harmful effects of addiction on the way the brain functions.

GROUP THERAPY

The types of therapy described in the previous sections can all be undertaken on an individual basis, but group therapy is also commonly used in addiction treatment. In fact, group therapy is often considered to be particularly well suited to addiction. Some of the benefits include:

- *Peer support (and peer pressure)*. Group members typically encourage each other's recovery efforts, reject excuses and denial, give each other helpful feedback, and share tips and strategies for avoiding substance use.
- *A sense of community*. Group participation reduces individual members' sense of isolation and helps them practice social skills they may have lost while they were using. This practice can also make them better at interacting with their family.
- *Information*. Members who are new to recovery often find what they learn from others in groups to be very educational.
- *Structure and discipline*. People whose lives are in chaos are often helped by the limitations, consequences, and responsibilities of participating in a group.
- *Friends*. Group members sometimes form relationships that continue outside the group setting.
- *Hope*. Addicts are able to witness the recovery of others and interact with people in long-term recovery, which can be inspiring.

Groups vary in their focus. Some are more educational, some prioritize emotional and practical support, and some follow a cognitive-behavioral model or focus heavily on relapse-prevention skills.

Group therapy is different from Twelve-Step and other support groups, and the two are not substitutes for each other. Group therapy sessions are led by trained professionals who apply psychotherapeutic techniques, whereas support groups tend to be led by the members themselves and focus more on the traditions and philosophy of the organization. Many people go to both group therapy and Twelve-Step or other meetings and derive distinct benefits from each.

27

Drugs That Treat Alcohol Abuse

There is no drug that can cure alcoholism, but there are several drugs that can make it easier for an alcoholic to stop drinking.

Three drugs have been specifically approved by the U.S. Food and Drug Administration for the treatment of alcoholism, and these drugs are generally available in other countries as well. Additionally, some drugs that are used primarily for other purposes may also be helpful to alcoholics.

The three main drugs take different approaches to the problem. Disulfiram (Antabuse) is designed to make alcoholics sick if they consume alcohol. Naltrexone (Revia, Vivitrol) neutralizes the effects of alcohol, so alcoholics stop experiencing a "benefit" from using it. And acamprosate (Campral) alleviates the cravings that alcoholics typically experience when they stop drinking.

Again, these drugs can *help* a person stop abusing alcohol, but they're not a cure in and of themselves. They're commonly prescribed to assist people in getting over the initial hurdle of quitting, although many people continue taking them for years afterward. In general, combining these drugs with additional forms of treatment, such as therapy and support groups, is considered more effective than simply taking the drugs alone in addressing underlying problems and supporting long-term recovery.

DISULFIRAM (ANTABUSE)

Antabuse is the oldest drug for alcoholism, having been used since the 1940s. It makes people sick if they consume alcohol, even in very small quantities. Thus, it basically "forces" alcoholics to stop drinking because they experience genuine suffering if they do.

Antabuse works by blocking an enzyme in the body that breaks down alcohol. Because the enzyme stops working, people who drink while taking the drug experience symptoms similar to those of a hangover, only much more intense. These may include nausea and vomiting, headaches, chest pain, blurred vision, mental confusion, sweating, breathing difficulty, heart palpitations, and anxiety. Anyone who has combined alcohol and Antabuse will tell you that it is not a fun time.

Used as directed, Antabuse *will* stop an alcoholic from drinking (although some alcoholics are tempted to "test" whether the drug actually works, usually with a very unpleasant result). The problem is that Antabuse won't stop an alcoholic from having cravings, and it won't solve the underlying psychological issues that caused the person to become an alcoholic in the first place. As a result, there is a very great tendency for alcoholics to simply stop using it.

Antabuse works best in a controlled setting, such as a clinic, where it's administered by someone else and the alcoholic doesn't have to choose each day whether to take the pill. It can also work where a family member is willing to supervise the alcoholic in taking the medication. However, a determined alcoholic can often still find a way to stop. For instance, there have been many cases where an alcoholic has only pretended to swallow the pill and spat it out later.

Antabuse is most effective where an alcoholic is highly motivated to quit but needs some additional help. As one alcoholic put it, "With Antabuse, I don't have to decide to stay sober 24 hours a day. I just have to decide to stay sober for 10 seconds each morning."

Antabuse users have to be careful because the medication is so sensitive that it can react to tiny amounts of alcohol found in cold remedies, mouthwash, sauces, desserts, and even some perfumes. Also, liver enzymes need to be monitored because the drug can have a toxic effect on the liver in a small number of cases.

NALTREXONE

Naltrexone works by blocking certain receptors in the brain that cause people to feel pleasure when they drink alcohol. As a result, alcohol becomes less pleasurable, and alcoholics may experience less desire for it. It is sold under the trade names Revia and Depade.

Unlike Antabuse, naltrexone won't definitely stop alcoholics from drinking, but it can be helpful in making it easier to quit. Many alcoholics experience a dramatic drop in cravings.

Like Antabuse, though, naltrexone works only if alcoholics keep taking it, and there's a tendency for alcoholics to stop taking it so they can once again experience the "high" they get from drinking.

One solution to this problem is to take naltrexone in the form of a monthly injection rather than a daily pill. In this way, the alcoholic has to decide to take the drug only once a month rather than once a day. The monthly injection is available under the trade name Vivitrol.

Naltrexone can cause health problems if it's taken by people who are pregnant or have liver or kidney damage.

ACAMPROSATE (CAMPRAL)

Campral is designed to reduce cravings in alcoholics who are not currently drinking. It does this by stimulating certain neurotransmitters in the brain.

Campral is typically prescribed for people who have gone without alcohol for a week or two, to make it easier for them to handle cravings and avoid relapse.

Unlike naltrexone, Campral won't stop people who drink from feeling drunk; in fact, it generally has no effect at all on alcoholics who are actively drinking. It also won't help with immediate withdrawal symptoms, which is why it isn't usually prescribed until alcoholics have been detoxed and have the immediate effects of alcohol out of their system.

OTHER DRUGS

Topiramate (Topamax) is an epilepsy drug, but it has been used in some cases for alcoholics. It works similarly to Campral in that it reduces cravings, but there is also evidence that it can help with certain non-craving withdrawal symptoms such as anxiety and depression.

Ondansetron (Zofran) is used primarily to reduce nausea and vomiting during cancer treatments. However, it may also help reduce alcohol cravings, primarily by affecting the brain's serotonin levels.

Other drugs that have shown at least some likelihood of helping alcoholics reduce the desire to drink include varenicline (a drug used to help people stop smoking, sold as Chantix and Champix) and gabapentin (used for seizures and nerve pain and sold as Neurontin, among other names).

DRUG TREATMENTS AND THE TWELVE STEPS

Some controversy exists as to whether drug treatments such as those in this chapter are compatible with Twelve-Step programs. In the case of drug treatments for *opioids*, the Narcotics Anonymous group has taken the position that such treatments may be helpful in giving up an addiction but that addicts should ultimately strive to be free of them in order to be completely "clean and sober." (See Chapter 28 for more details.) Alcoholics Anonymous, however, does not take an official position on drug treatments.

AA is a decentralized organization, and some individual AA groups have been known to discourage members from relying on drugs to get over alcoholism. However, AA's "Twelve Traditions" warns that the group should never take a position on any public controversy, and at least one official AA publication warns members that, whatever they may personally think of a drug such as Antabuse, they should not suggest to others that AA *itself* has an official position on it. (See "Traditions Checklist from the AA Grapevine," *www.aa.org/assets/en_US/smf-131_en.pdf.*)

• • • • • • • **28** • • • • • •

Drugs That Treat
Opioid Abuse

U nfortunately, no drugs have been developed yet that are highly effective at treating addictions to stimulants, depressants, or marijuana. These addictions are commonly treated through some combination of detox, psychotherapy, and support groups.

However, a number of drugs are now being used to treat opioid addiction. This chapter will discuss them.

In understanding how these drugs work, it's useful to understand how opioids themselves work. Opioids, including many prescription painkillers and heroin, attach to certain proteins in the brain and elsewhere called "opioid receptors." They activate these receptors, which results in the alleviation of pain—and also a release of dopamine, which is where the addictive tendency comes from.

A drug that attaches to opioid receptors and fully activates them is called a full agonist. There are other drugs that attach to opioid receptors but only partially activate them. These are known as partial agonists. Finally, there are drugs that attach to opioid receptors, do not activate them at all, and block other drugs from attaching to them and activating them. These are known as opioid *antagonists*.

With drug treatments for opioid abuse, there are two main strategies. The first strategy is to give addicts full or partial agonists that will satisfy their cravings for an opioid response, but not get them "high" or trigger the addiction cycle. The second strategy is to give addicts antagonists that will block any addictive drugs from working.

Here's a look at the most common drugs used for treatment of opioid addiction.

METHADONE

Methadone is the best-known drug for the treatment of heroin addiction, having been around in the United States since the 1940s. Methadone is a full opioid agonist, meaning that it attaches to opioid receptors and fully activates them—so it largely eliminates cravings, but it doesn't produce a high. It can be used to manage withdrawal symptoms; it can also be used as a long-term substitute for heroin and other drugs in what's known as a methadone maintenance program.

Because methadone can be dangerous if misused—you can actually overdose on methadone—it is typically administered daily in a controlled setting by a pharmacist or other professional. Many places specialize in this type of treatment and are called methadone clinics.

A lot of people who are addicted to heroin or other opioids have made major improvements in their lives through a methadone maintenance program. And while methadone typically isn't covered by insurance (except for Medicaid), the daily doses are relatively inexpensive.

Nevertheless, methadone has its share of critics. Some people believe that long-term methadone use really just amounts to substituting one addiction for another and that people become enslaved to methadone in somewhat the same way that they were enslaved to heroin. These people often advocate weaning users off methadone by gradually reducing doses over a period of months.

This can work in some cases. However, because methadone is a full agonist, it's also possible that cravings will return. Methadone advocates often claim that weaning people off methadone only increases the chances that they will end up going back to more dangerous street drugs instead.

Other critics have pointed out that methadone can be a highly inconvenient form of treatment. For instance, not everyone lives near a methadone clinic, so some people have a very long drive every single day to get treatment—which can interfere with work schedules and other life responsibilities.

Also, standing in line every day at a methadone clinic with other former heroin users can make it very difficult for addicts to escape the "milieu" they knew when they were getting high, which in itself can lead to temptations to relapse. And some drug dealers have been known to prey on people near methadone clinics, knowing that the occasional urge to relapse makes them potential customers.

NALTREXONE

Unlike methadone, which is an opioid agonist, naltrexone is an opioid *antagonist*. It works by blocking other drugs from activating opioid receptors in the brain. As a result, other opioid drugs become less pleasurable, and addicts may experience less desire for them. However, the drug doesn't do anything to reduce the physiological cravings resulting from withdrawal.

Naltrexone is the only drug that is prescribed for both alcoholics and drug addicts. The main problem with the drug for opioid use is the same as the main problem for alcohol use—it relies on people taking it every day, and since it doesn't reduce cravings, people may be tempted to stop taking it so they can once again feel the pleasurable effects of the drug.

As with alcohol, a solution to this problem is to take naltrexone in the form of a monthly injection rather than a daily pill. The monthly injection is available under the trade name Vivitrol.

Another problem with naltrexone is that addicts must have successfully detoxed and then remained abstinent for a week or more before using it—and many addicts aren't able to get to this point. (Using naltrexone without having detoxed can result in severe withdrawal symptoms.)

Naltrexone can also cause health problems if taken by people who are pregnant or have liver or kidney damage.

BUPRENORPHINE

Buprenorphine has a double effect. On the one hand, it's a partial agonist, so it satisfies some drug cravings without getting the person high. But it also works in some ways as an antagonist, so it blocks other drugs from having an effect.

Buprenorphine is a tablet that allows the drug to be absorbed through the cheek or under the tongue. It's sold under the brand name Subutex.

The main problem with buprenorphine is that, since it's a partial agonist, it can create some of the same pleasurable effects as prescription painkillers and street drugs. After a while, it was discovered that some people were crushing their buprenorphine tablets and then snorting them or injecting them, which can intensify the effects and create a drug high.

As a result, buprenorphine is now available in a long-term injectable form, with the brand names Probuphine and Sublocade. It comes in one-week, four-week, and six-month versions. This eliminates the risk that tablets will be misused or that addicts will stop taking them.

SUBOXONE

Suboxone is another solution to the "buprenorphine problem." It's a combination of buprenorphine and a drug called naloxone, which is a derivative of naltrexone and an opioid antagonist. (Naloxone is sold under the trade name Narcan and is also used to reverse overdoses of heroin and other opioids, as discussed in Chapter 20.)

The addition of naloxone is meant to prevent people who misuse buprenorphine from experiencing a high. The drug was also reformulated as a dissolvable film to further prevent it from being misused.

Although Suboxone is the most common trade name, the drug combination is also available under the names Zubsolv and Bunavail.

Like methadone, Suboxone can be used for long periods in a maintenance program to keep people from using other drugs. Many people have consistently stayed clean while on a Suboxone regimen.

The risk of overdose is much lower with Suboxone than with methadone. For this reason, Suboxone is less tightly controlled, and users can pick up a prescription at a pharmacy and take the drug at home rather than having to go to a clinic every day to have it administered. This is a very big advantage.

There are some drawbacks to Suboxone, however. One is that, since the drug is a partial agonist, if addicts suddenly stop using it they may experience significant withdrawal symptoms. People can gradually wean themselves off Suboxone, but it often takes a very long time. Another problem is that it can be very dangerous for Suboxone users to drink alcohol or take benzodiazepines. Yet another problem is that, if people who are *not* addicted to opioids get their hands on Suboxone and use it, they can actually become addicted to it—after all, it's a partial agonist.

In fact, Suboxone is frequently sold on the black market, where it has the nicknames "sub" and "box." The fact that the drug is more easily available than methadone has exacerbated this problem.

A 2018 study sponsored by the National Institute on Drug Abuse compared the results of treatment using Suboxone and Vivitrol (a monthly naltrexone injection). The six-month relapse rates for addicts using the two drugs were roughly the same, with the Vivitrol rate being very slightly lower. However, Suboxone still "won" in the end because Vivitrol requires addicts to detox and then remain abstinent for a week before using it—and a significant number of the Vivitrol test subjects weren't able to do so. Thus, many people in the Vivitrol group dropped out without ever having received the shot.

Suboxone works best when it's prescribed by a doctor who is an addiction specialist and when it is combined with other forms of treatment and regular drug screenings to make sure the person isn't abusing the drug or, worse, mixing it with benzodiazepines.

Unfortunately, in many places today Suboxone is prescribed at cash-only clinics that do little in the way of counseling or drug testing. People can sometimes misuse the drug by showing up at multiple clinics and getting multiple prescriptions, a practice known as "box shopping."

DRUG TREATMENTS AND THE TWELVE STEPS

Some controversy exists over whether the drug treatments described in this chapter are compatible with Twelve-Step programs. Some individual Twelve-Step groups support the use of these treatments, while others believe that addicts who are receiving them are still using drugs and are therefore not truly clean and sober.

Narcotics Anonymous, the largest Twelve-Step group for drug addicts, takes no official position on the value of medication-assisted treatments. (See Chapter 30 for more information on this group.) However, the NA organization emphasizes that it believes the proper way to treat addiction is through complete abstinence and application of the

Twelve-Step principles, and therefore it advocates that members should strive to ultimately live free of drug treatments even if they need such treatments temporarily to help in their recovery. As an example, NA's central book, called the *Basic Text*, offers the story of an addict who was on methadone for 10 months before finally giving it up and becoming "clean."

The NA organization notes that individual NA meetings are largely autonomous and that some are very open to drug treatments, some are occasionally critical, and some limit the participation of people who are receiving such help. It suggests that addicts who are recovering with the use of drug treatments seek out meetings where they will be the most welcome. (For the full text of the NA position, see "Narcotics Anonymous and Persons Receiving Medication-Assisted Treatment," *www. na.org/admin/include/spaw2/uploads/pdf/pr/2306_NA_PRMAT_1021. pdf.*)

In response to the NA's stance, a group called Medication Assisted Recovery Anonymous has been formed to offer a Twelve-Step program for people who believe that abstaining from opioids with the help of drug treatments is a fully valid form of recovery.

29

Does Alcoholics Anonymous Actually Work?

Does Alcoholics Anonymous work? Yes—sometimes.

AA has helped a lot of people achieve long-term sobriety. A significant number of people will tell you that they owe the very fact that they are still alive to the program.

On the other hand, many people go to a few AA meetings, don't like them, and leave. And many people go to meetings frequently and practice the Twelve Steps as best they can, but relapse over and over again.

There have been a number of attempts to quantify how often AA succeeds, and the results of these studies vary considerably. A few of them suggest that the success rate is quite low. Some doctors who advocate psychotherapy as a primary treatment have cited these latter statistics in an attempt to debunk AA and prove that it doesn't work.

The problem is that, for a number of reasons, it's extremely difficult to establish statistically exactly what AA's success rate is. For instance, since addiction has no cure and can at best be managed as a long-term chronic condition, what constitutes "success"? A person who never drinks again obviously counts as a success, but what about a person who is able to lead a generally productive life despite occasional relapses? What about people who die as a result of long-term complications of alcoholism but were able through AA to extend their lives by a year or two?

Many people who go to AA are also receiving other types of treatment, such as therapy or prescription drugs. How can it be determined how much of their success is due to AA as opposed to these other treatments?

In addition, since AA has no particular rules about how often one must attend meetings or how one should approach the Twelve Steps, it's hard to establish exactly who should "count" in determining the success rate. Many people attend meetings only sporadically or infrequently and don't engage seriously in other aspects of the program. If they keep drinking, has AA failed?

Moreover, a significant number of people who attend AA meetings don't do so voluntarily. Some have been pressured by a family member or employer. Others attend as part of a court diversion program following a drunk-driving or drug offense, which means they're not necessarily there because they genuinely want to get better, but simply because they want to avoid going to jail. If these people *don't* get better, is it because AA didn't work?

In the end, it's probably meaningless to try to quantify how successful AA is. What we know is that it definitely works for some people, and it's a resource that should be considered seriously—especially since all it typically asks for is a small voluntary donation for coffee and refreshments, which means it's a whole lot cheaper than psychotherapy or an inpatient rehab program.

Because AA can be a valuable resource, and because a large number of rehab programs are built on the Twelve-Step model, it's worth explaining the program in some detail—how it started, how it works, and what actually happens in AA.

HOW IT STARTED

AA began in the mid-1930s as an informal group founded by a stock speculator, Bill Wilson, and a doctor, Bob Smith. (The two are known within AA as Bill W. and Dr. Bob.) After the two men achieved sobriety, they began trying to help other alcoholics do the same, convinced that recovery was possible through reliance on a "higher power" and the support of fellow alcoholics. The two eventually developed a program of Twelve Steps, which AA members try to follow as a path to recovery.

By 1939, the pair claimed to have helped more than 100 alcoholics attain sobriety. At that point they published a book, called *Alcoholics Anonymous: The Story of How More Than One Hundred Men Have Recovered from Alcoholism*. The name of their organization, Alcoholics Anonymous, was derived from the title of the book. The book is still in print and forms the basis for much of what occurs in AA. Within the program, it is referred to as the Big Book.

Today there are more than 100,000 AA groups worldwide. These groups are largely independent, self-supporting through small donations, and run by the members themselves. There is a small central organization that supports itself through donations and printing books and literature, but AA is generally nonhierarchical, and the central organization exercises little if any control over the individual groups.

An important document called the "Twelve Traditions" outlines much of the mission and purpose of AA. Among other things, it states that AA exists solely as a forum for members to help each other and themselves and should never endorse a political position, lend its name to any other organization, or take part in public controversies. It also warns against most types of public marketing and promotion.

THE TWELVE STEPS

The Twelve Steps form the core of AA and of many similar programs that are known as Twelve-Step programs. Broadly speaking, the steps describe the experiences of the organization's earliest members in acknowledging that they couldn't control their drinking, giving themselves over to a higher power, admitting their faults, and making amends to others. The steps are very brief—less than a sentence each. They can't be reproduced here due to international copyright law, but you can find them on the AA website at *www.aa.org/assets/en_US/smf-121_en.pdf*. It's worth taking a moment to read them.

SPONSORS AND WORKING THE STEPS

AA members are encouraged to "work the steps" by applying them to their lives. This is usually done in conjunction with a sponsor.

A sponsor is a more experienced AA member, usually one who has achieved a lengthy period of sustained sobriety. The sponsor's chief role is to help the member work through the steps and to be available in a crisis if the member needs help avoiding the temptation to relapse. New AA members are often encouraged to choose someone as a temporary sponsor, who can be available to them while they search for someone with whom they feel more personally comfortable as a permanent sponsor. It's traditional for men to choose male sponsors and for women to choose female sponsors.

"Working the steps" is an amorphous process. Some people go through them very quickly; some take years. Some go through them over and over again. There is no formal procedure, no timeline, and no graduation. The steps are considered a type of discipline that people can keep referring back to as they gradually change their addictive lifestyle.

In actual practice, many people go to AA meetings regularly, sometimes for very long periods, without ever having a sponsor or formally working the steps.

WHAT HAPPENS AT MEETINGS

Meetings typically last about an hour (some last an hour and a half) and are run by a chairperson. The chairperson is a member who has temporarily volunteered for the role.

Meetings take several forms, but they have a typical structure. There are a number of standard practices at the beginning (or sometimes at the end), which include announcements and welcoming of new attendees and visitors. Certain passages from the Big Book are often read, including a section called How It Works and what are known as the Promises. The Twelve Traditions may also be read, along with something called the Preamble and possibly guidelines for the group. At some point a collection is taken.

The core of an AA meeting consists of going around the room and giving each member a chance to speak in turn. Often a passage from the Big Book will be read, and members will be asked to speak in a way that responds to the subject of that passage.

Members are asked to limit their speaking time so that everyone in the room has a chance to speak. (Typically, the limit is about three minutes.) Members who speak usually begin by saying, "I'm Bob, and I'm an alcoholic." Everyone responds, "Hi, Bob." When the speaker is finished, everyone says, "Thanks, Bob." Members who don't want to speak can pass.

A key rule in meetings is the avoidance of "crosstalk," which means that members do not interrupt one another and do not refer directly to what someone else said or try to give that person advice. Because of this rule, members generally never have to fear that their feelings or ideas will be commented on or criticized or that others will adopt a posture of superiority toward them. On the other hand, some people are frustrated by the rule because they would genuinely like discussion and feedback about their situation.

Some meetings are speaker meetings. A person will be invited at the beginning to speak at some length on a topic, and afterward members will be encouraged to address their comments to the topic.

Some meetings are step-study meetings. These are limited to a discussion of one of the steps. Speaking at these meetings is usually limited to members who have worked that particular step.

"Open" meetings are open to anyone; "closed" meetings are limited to alcoholics, and guests and observers are not invited. Some meetings are limited by membership and are open only to, for example, women, men, young people, or members of the LGBTQ community.

Meetings typically close with the "serenity prayer," attributed to the American theologian Reinhold Niebuhr. It goes: "God, grant me the serenity to accept the things I cannot change, courage to change the things I can, and wisdom to know the difference."

HOW DOES IT WORK?

AA takes a fundamentally different approach from that of psychotherapy or drug therapy.

Psychotherapy treats addiction primarily as a *psychological* problem, one that can be alleviated by helping people achieve a better understanding of their inner feelings and motivations. Drug therapy treats addiction primarily as a *biochemical* problem, one that can be alleviated by adjusting the person's brain chemistry.

AA, on the other hand, treats addiction primarily as a *spiritual* problem, one that can be alleviated by causing people to take a different view of their place in the universe.

Many addicts are in denial about their condition. They continue to believe, despite all evidence to the contrary, that they can control their disease and moderate their consumption. The first step in AA is to give up this belief—to accept that one is powerless over the disease.

Accepting powerlessness—giving up ego control—makes way for the acceptance of something larger than oneself—a higher power, however one might conceive such a thing. By giving up denial and control, agreeing that one is powerless, and humbly and unflinchingly acknowledging all one's faults, one is able to undergo a spiritual transformation in which one no longer needs to rely on alcohol to feel worthwhile and important.

Many people use alcohol and drugs as a way of battling their underlying feelings of anxiety, inadequacy, and lack of self-worth. AA says, in effect, that it is pointless to try to fight these feelings—that one should instead *embrace* them. Compared to the larger universe—or higher power—we are *all* inadequate; we are all failures to some degree. But that doesn't mean that we can't be good people. The key is humility—the first step in becoming a better person is acknowledging that we are not perfect. By embracing one's limitations, one no longer needs to rely on a substance to forget about them.

Another aspect of humility is taking responsibility. The Twelve Steps encourage people to take a "moral inventory" and accept responsibility for their actions and decisions. Of course, no one can control all the external circumstances of life, but people can control the ways they react to them. Accepting responsibility for the things that one can control tends to correct the natural tendency of addicts to blame other people and situations for all their problems.

That's the underlying theory of the Twelve Steps. The other aspect of AA is the meetings. The meetings are useful from an educational point of view because members can learn from one another's coping mechanisms. But more than that, the meetings give members an opportunity to help one another. As you might imagine, helping others is usually the last thing that people in the throes of active addiction have on their minds. Helping others takes you out of yourself and is an antidote to the common addictive tendency toward self-centeredness and self-focus. (Indeed, a study led by a Harvard Medical School professor showed that attending AA meetings can significantly reduce symptoms of depression.)

One thing you notice if you go to a lot of AA meetings is that many of the people there do seem extraordinarily humble. It really does seem as if some of them have undergone a spiritual transformation.

But again, does this theory work *to solve addiction?* Obviously, it works very well for some people. But for whatever reason, other people don't seem to get much benefit out of it.

One criticism of AA's philosophy is that it might in some cases be directly contrary to the goals of psychotherapy. In many forms of therapy, the goal is not to persuade addicts that they're powerless, but to persuade them that they can in fact have control over the disease and to empower them with tools and techniques to resist cravings and make better decisions on their own. This might explain why some therapists take a skeptical approach to Twelve-Step programs.

IS ALCOHOLICS ANONYMOUS A RELIGION?

A number of people are put off by AA's religious overtones. It's possible to be a member of AA without participating in any of the religious aspects of it, but those aspects are nevertheless built into the structure of the organization.

The exact relationship between AA and religion is somewhat difficult to pin down.

On the one hand, the founders of AA, Bill W. and Dr. Bob, were members of the Oxford Group, a nondenominational religious assembly modeled on early Christianity. At the very beginning, the founders worked with a specifically Christian model, although they increasingly departed from it as they began to form what became AA.

The Twelve Steps contain explicitly religious language. Five of the steps refer to God, and the eleventh step involves prayer. The goal of the group is described as gaining sobriety through a "spiritual awakening," and meetings usually close with the serenity prayer and sometimes the "Our Father" or Lord's Prayer.

On the other hand, the group has no ties at all to any specific religious group or sect. It welcomes people of all religions and people who have no religion. Although the Twelve-Step language refers to God, it defines God simply as a higher power (or "power greater than ourselves") and invites people to think of this power in any way they want to—it refers to God "as we understood Him," and no particular type of understanding is expected or provided.

While it's true that AA meetings often occur in church basements, that's not because AA has ties to a particular church. Rather, churches often have space to rent during the week and may see renting or providing space to AA as part of their mission to help the disadvantaged.

Overall, a good way to view AA might be that it is an organization with Christian roots whose philosophy and mode of expression have been adapted over time to an increasingly secular and religiously diverse population.

Also, each of the more than 100,000 AA groups operates autonomously. As a result, different groups take on different characteristics depending on their particular membership. At some, religion is discussed freely and frequently. Some groups make a special effort to avoid any discussion of religion. And most are somewhere in the middle, with members occasionally mentioning spirituality but most of the focus staying on more everyday practical concerns.

People who like AA in general but are uncomfortable with the religious aspects of it can shop around for a meeting that better suits their needs. There is even a group within AA called We Agnostics. We Agnostics meetings operate exactly like AA meetings, except that there are no prayers and talk about religion is discouraged. Another group, called Secular AA, offers a number of meetings online.

More information on finding AA meetings can be found in the Resources at the back of the book.

• • • • • • • 30 • • • • • • • •

AA-Type Groups
for Addictions
Other Than Alcohol

As Alcoholics Anonymous has grown in popularity, it has inspired a large number of other Twelve-Step groups dedicated to different types of addiction.

AA, of course, was founded specifically to help alcoholics. The very first of the Twelve Steps requires members to admit that they are "powerless over alcohol." Over time, however, AA groups began to find that a growing number of drug addicts were showing up at AA meetings. This created a dilemma—should they be allowed to join?

AA wanted to help such people, but it feared that becoming an organization dedicated to all types of addictions would dilute its mission. It also worried that, while alcoholics have a special bond of understanding with each other that makes the meetings work, such a bond might not exist as strongly between alcoholics and drug addicts.

AA's solution was that it would allow its basic principles—the Twelve Steps and Twelve Traditions—to be used by any other group that wanted to do so, including groups dedicated to drug addiction. AA would cooperate with such groups but not affiliate with them. This gave rise to Narcotics Anonymous, or NA, the first and largest of the "alternative" Twelve-Step groups.

NA is extremely similar to AA in practice, with one of the few differences being that the word "alcohol" in the first step is changed to "addiction." Of course, another difference is that AA members deal with only a single substance of choice—alcohol—whereas NA members may have dozens of different substances of choice.

Rather than the AA Big Book, NA uses something called the *Basic Text,* which has been revised many times over the years. The NA organization has published several other books, including *It Works: How and Why* and *Living Clean: The Journey Continues.*

There are more than 25,000 NA groups worldwide. While that's a very large number, it is dwarfed by the number of AA groups. As a result, in any given locale, there are typically a lot more AA meetings than NA meetings. Because of this, and because the structure of the groups' meetings is so similar, many drug addicts who want to attend more frequent meetings still end up going to AA meetings. Some AA groups are more accepting of drug addicts than others, so drug addicts who want to attend AA meetings might want to try several groups to find the ones where they feel most comfortable.

The official AA policy is that drug addicts are welcome at open AA meetings, but closed AA meetings are for alcoholics only and drug addicts are not invited. Despite this official policy, though, in practice some closed AA meetings are willing to accept drug addicts. Of course, people who are addicted to *both* alcohol and drugs are officially welcome at both open and closed AA and NA meetings.

In recent years, a number of newer Twelve-Step programs have arisen that are dedicated to specific drugs. These include Marijuana Anonymous, Cocaine Anonymous, Heroin Anonymous, and Crystal Meth Anonymous. Some of these groups have developed their own literature, while others simply borrow from AA publications. There are also groups for process addictions, including Gamblers Anonymous, Overeaters Anonymous, Spenders Anonymous, and Sex Addicts Anonymous. A group called Dual Recovery Anonymous is for people who have both an addiction and a separate emotional or psychiatric illness. And a group called Medication Assisted Recovery Anonymous focuses on opioid addicts who are using methadone or other drug treatments. (These treatments are discussed in Chapter 28.)

More information on all these groups can be found in the Resources at the back of the book.

31

Alternative Support Groups for People Who Don't Like AA

Addicts who want to attend a support group but don't particularly like AA or other Twelve-Step meetings (because of their religious aspects or for other reasons) should know that there are various alternatives.

What follows is a list of other support groups for addicts. A major problem with these groups is that they're much smaller than AA or NA, so it might be difficult to find meetings nearby or to find meetings that occur as frequently as addicts would like. (Of course, there's nothing stopping addicts from attending meetings of these groups *in addition to* going to AA or NA meetings.)

SMART Recovery is perhaps the leading alternative to AA and NA. It is explicitly secular and does not use the Twelve Steps. SMART (which stands for Self-Management and Recovery Training) is based on cognitive and behavioral psychology and tries to offer practical tools for addicts to use to change their behavior. Unlike AA, the group doesn't believe that addiction is a spiritual sickness or that addicts need to acknowledge that they are powerless over their disease. In fact, SMART believes addicts *do* have the power to change their circumstances simply by changing the way they think about them. The main focus is on understanding why addicts make the choices they do and how to change addicts' mindsets so that they can make better decisions.

SMART meetings differ from AA meetings in that there is often a lively back-and-forth discussion, as opposed to each person speaking in turn and being discouraged from responding to anyone else. The emphasis is on problem solving and finding better ways to deal with specific issues that arise in people's lives, usually by looking at what causes people to take the actions they do and what other ways of thinking they might use instead. Participants sometimes role-play situations to explore alternative ways of responding.

SMART meetings are free, although a small donation is requested. SMART also offers young people's groups, online meetings, message boards, and chat rooms.

Women for Sobriety was founded in the 1970s by Jean Kirkpatrick, a sociologist who claims she overcame her alcoholism by changing her negative thought patterns. In contrast to AA's focus on humility, WFS emphasizes empowerment and replacing lonely and depressed thoughts with a sense of self-worth and emotional growth. The group is limited to women, believing that women's addiction problems often stem from gender-specific emotional issues and should be addressed differently from those of men.

Secular Organizations for Sobriety, or SOS, was founded in the 1980s by James Christopher, an alcoholic who tried AA but felt uncomfortable with the idea of turning his life over to a higher power. SOS emphasizes self-reliance and personal responsibility. The group's focus is on what it calls the sobriety priority—the belief that for a person to get well, sobriety must always be his or her number-one concern in life.

LifeRing Secular Recovery is an offshoot group of SOS that was created after members disagreed about SOS's form of organization.

Celebrate Recovery is for people who believe that AA isn't religious enough. The group is part of the Saddleback Church run by pastor Rick Warren (the author of the book *The Purpose Driven Life*), and takes a more explicitly Christ-centered approach to the Twelve Steps. Celebrate Recovery chapters exist at many evangelical churches.

Moderation Management is a nonreligious group that rejects the idea that drinkers must engage in total abstinence to get well. Members are encouraged to abstain for 30 days and then set reasonable drinking guidelines and limits. The group believes that this approach can reduce harm for people who don't feel ready to give up drinking altogether.

DO THEY WORK?

There's not much hard evidence on the effectiveness of alternative support groups in comparison to Twelve-Step groups.

One study published in 2018 in the *Journal of Substance Abuse Treatment* compared long-term relapse rates for alcoholics in AA, Women for Sobriety, SMART Recovery, and LifeRing. The study found that relapse rates were somewhat higher in LifeRing and SMART Recovery. However, it also found that people who joined LifeRing and SMART Recovery were less committed to total lifelong abstinence as a treatment goal than people who joined AA were. Thus, it's not clear that the LifeRing and SMART Recovery approaches are less *effective* than that of AA; there might simply be a self-selection process whereby people who are more committed to total abstinence in the first place are more likely to join AA than the other groups.

More information on alternative support groups can be found in the Resources at the back of the book.

When an Addict Has Other Mental Health Problems

There's a very significant overlap between addiction and other forms of mental illness. Understanding the relationship between the two can be extremely important in aiding an addict's recovery.

According to U.S. government figures from 2014, some 20.2 million Americans suffer from a substance use disorder. Of those, some 7.9 million (or 39 percent) also have some other form of mental illness, and 2.3 million (or 11 percent) have a "serious" mental illness, meaning one that substantially limits a person's major life activities.

These figures, along with other studies, suggest that people with an addiction are far more likely than the general population to have another form of mental illness. Studies also show that there's a proportional relationship, meaning that the more severe a person's other mental illness is, the more likely it is that he or she will also have an addiction.

Mental illnesses that commonly coincide with addiction include depression, anxiety disorders, personality disorders, psychotic disorders, attention-deficit/hyperactivity disorder, and posttraumatic stress disorder. However, a number of other problems such as anorexia and obsessive–compulsive disorder are also found among addicts.

When people suffer from both an addiction and another mental illness, this is sometimes called a dual diagnosis, although the more contemporary term is "co-occurring disorders."

THE CHICKEN OR THE EGG?

It's often hard to tell which came first—the addiction or the co-occurring disorder. In some people, it appears that the other mental illness is the primary problem. The addiction may have arisen later, as the person attempted to self-medicate to cope with the underlying psychological disorder. But in others, the addiction is the primary issue. The other mental health problem may have developed as a result of the addiction's gradually interfering with the person's ability to cope. Finally, in some people it's difficult to tell which disorder is primary, and the two disorders are truly co-occurring.

HOW ARE THEY RELATED?

It's hard to say exactly how addiction and other mental disorders are related. Certainly there are some differences in how they arise. For instance, the biological mechanisms of addiction develop following repeated exposure to a substance, and therefore substance exposure is *necessary* for the problem to occur. This is not true for other mental illnesses and constitutes an important distinction.

That said, though, if you accept the stress–vulnerability model of mental illness (described in Chapter 4), there could be a connection in how the problems develop. This model views mental illness as a result of the interplay between biological and genetic susceptibility, coping mechanisms, and environmental stress factors. It's possible that some of the same genetic variants that make people susceptible to addiction might also make them susceptible to other mental illnesses, for instance. Also, to the extent that stress and poor coping mechanisms can trigger addiction, they may be able to trigger other mental illnesses as well.

Interestingly, people who are addicted to different substances tend to be more likely to have different mental illnesses. For instance, although antisocial personality disorder is rare, alcoholics are 21 times more likely to have it than the average person—whereas they are no more likely to have an anxiety disorder than the average person. On the other hand, a person with an anxiety disorder is twice as likely as the average person to develop an addiction of some sort.

One study has suggested that drug addicts are more likely than alcoholics to have an additional mental illness, although the figures are high for both groups.

It's also interesting to note that people with mental illnesses are more likely than the general population to use nicotine, although it varies by the type of mental illness. Among people with schizophrenia, the rate of smokers has been reported to be as high as 95 percent.

One thing that can be said for sure is that, in people with co-occurring disorders, the two disorders tend to make each other worse. A person with one disorder will automatically have more stress and fewer coping abilities and thus a much harder time dealing effectively with the other disorder.

INTEGRATED TREATMENT

For a long time, it was thought that addiction was a wholly separate problem from other mental illnesses. As a result, doctors tended to treat them separately and independently. This created a number of difficulties. A doctor treating one disorder, for instance, might prescribe a drug that made the other disorder worse or that negated or even interacted dangerously with a drug prescribed for the other disorder.

Drug addicts are often used to self-medicating their symptoms, so it was not uncommon for them to adjust the dosages of the medications prescribed for their other disorder on their own—which could make them ineffective or even cause health risks.

And some Twelve-Step groups were known to discourage members from taking their prescription medications for co-occurring disorders, claiming that taking drugs for an unrelated mental health problem meant that they weren't truly "clean and sober." (This, by the way, is not true. For an official AA publication debunking this claim, see *www. aa.org/assets/en_US/p-11_aamembersMedDrug.pdf*.)

As a result of these problems, most professionals today recommend integrated treatment—a course of care in which both problems are treated at the same time, either by the same professional or by different professionals working together as a team. This tends to produce better results because it takes both disorders and the relationship between them into account.

Integrated group therapy has also been developed, focusing on how to manage the interaction between multiple disorders. There are even groups for specific co-occurring disorders such as bipolar disorder and posttraumatic stress disorder.

ENABLING AND CO-OCCURRING DISORDERS

While most families of addicted loved ones eventually learn that enabling behavior is counterproductive, avoiding this kind of behavior can be much more complex when a loved one has a co-occurring disorder.

In such cases, the family is often tempted to take actions that would otherwise appear to be enabling so as to help the addict cope with or treat the other issue. For instance, many families keep close tabs on addicts to make sure they take medication for their other disorder rather than letting them experience the natural consequences of failing to do so. Families can also be more tempted to bail an addict out of problems or let an addicted child continue living at home when the addict's difficulty coping isn't "simply" a matter of coming to grips with an addiction.

This is a difficult dilemma. In general, families need to recognize that even addicts with other mental health issues eventually need to learn to make good decisions on their own and take responsibility for their actions. But with a co-occurring disorder, drawing the precise line between enabling and sensibly protecting can be extremely challenging.

V

WHAT TO EXPECT
IN RECOVERY

• • • • • • • **33** • • • • • • • •

What to Expect
in Early Recovery

There's no "official" definition of early recovery, but most professionals consider it to include the first year after someone becomes clean and sober. That's surprising to many people. A *full year*, and you're still just in "early" recovery? Yes. Addictions don't develop in a day, and recovery doesn't happen quickly either. It takes a lot of time. The biggest mistake that people make with early recovery—both addicts and their families—is to expect too much too soon.

Addicts sometimes feel a temporary rush of relief once the heavy alcohol or drug use starts to wear off. Sometimes the recovery process doesn't initially seem as bad as they had feared. They develop a dangerous overconfidence—a sense of "I've got this." (In AA, this is often referred to as "the pink cloud.") This overconfidence can cause them to miss meetings and treatments and expose themselves to situations full of temptations. The result is often relapse.

Family members sometimes assume that once addicts come back from detox or rehab they'll be "well" and everything will go back to normal. They expect them to handle all their old responsibilities and to be emotionally present to others as though nothing ever happened. These expectations can put a great deal of stress on addicts and undermine their recovery.

To get a better sense of early recovery, it's helpful to understand what's happening in the brain.

THIS IS YOUR BRAIN NO LONGER ON DRUGS

Addiction causes structural changes in the brain, both in the pleasure centers and in the prefrontal cortex. When a person goes through detox and gets past the immediate symptoms of withdrawal, those changes are still there. They don't simply disappear. The brain does have a marvelous ability to heal itself, but it happens gradually. It generally takes about three months for the prefrontal cortex to begin to return to something like its normal state. Until then, the decision-making scale is still heavily and unnaturally weighted toward using substances.

The first three months of sobriety are usually the most difficult period and the time when the risk of relapse is greatest. Addicts are still extremely fragile. Although they may not be actively using, their brain is still telling them that they should be, and it takes all their effort to resist the urges. (Although it's often financially out of the question, this is why many experts say that a minimum 90-day stay in a residential treatment program is ideal.)

Healing in the pleasure-center part of the brain takes even longer. While addicts gradually get back much of their decision-making faculties after three months, the emotional impulses to use remain strong. Because dopamine is still not being regulated properly, the addict who isn't getting a drug-related dopamine fix often continues to experience a significant happiness deficit.

The scientific name for this is post-acute withdrawal syndrome, or PAWS. The typical symptoms of PAWS include anxiety, irritability, mood swings, tiredness, depression, inability to concentrate, and sleep problems. PAWS can last a year or longer, and the desire to escape the symptoms of PAWS is a major cause of relapse.

RELEARNING EVERYTHING

Addiction is a process whereby people become completely dependent on a substance. Whatever problems they might experience in life, the substance is the answer. It's the self-medication that makes them feel like they can cope and go on. As a result, when an addict goes into treatment and gives up the substance, it's not like a healthy person giving up sweets. It's like a person having to learn all over again how to handle every aspect of life in a different way. Some people have compared it to a right-handed person having to learn to do everything with the left hand. It's possible, but it takes a tremendous amount of getting used to.

If an addict is to succeed, then the entire focus of life in early recovery has to be on staying clean and sober. It's not just the top priority; it's the *only* priority. Taking your eyes off the ball is not an option.

For this reason, most professionals recommend against people in early recovery taking on heavy job responsibilities or engaging in new pursuits that demand a lot of attention. For example, one study showed that single women who become romantically involved with someone in the first three months of recovery are five times more likely to relapse than single women who don't.

WHAT IT'S LIKE FOR FAMILIES

The reality of early recovery can be extremely difficult for family members. After all, when addicts are using, family members typically experience them as acting selfishly, putting their own needs above those of others, and focusing all their attention on substance use. In effect, during early recovery, that's all still true—addicts have to focus exclusively on themselves and on their own needs to stay away from drugs.

Family members often feel a tremendous letdown. They wanted to get back the person they used to know—but they still haven't succeeded. Instead, they may be living with someone who is moody, irritable, depressed, and self-absorbed and probably not able to fully take on all the responsibilities of his or her old life.

It often takes about six months of recovery before a person begins to spontaneously express interest in and concern for other family members' well-being. At first this happens sporadically. It may be a full year before it begins to occur on a regular basis. What's happening is that the addict is gradually learning the process of living without addictive substances. At first, this requires 100 percent of his or her attention. As the addict gradually gets used to a new way of living and develops greater mastery of the skills of being clean and sober, he or she has more mental attention available to respond to other people's needs.

The problem for family members during early recovery is that all the emotions that they are likely to have felt during the person's active addiction—anger, hurt, obsession, and so on—are still there. They don't simply vanish once the addict returns home. As an example, families often want desperately for addicts to apologize for their behavior and to acknowledge the family's pain and all they had to go through. At last, they think, the addict will finally pay attention to them and make it up to them for what they endured. But unfortunately, paying attention to others' emotional needs is a skill that most addicts will regain only slowly over time.

Continued obsession with the addict can manifest itself in a number of ways, such as an extreme fear of relapse. Some families have been known to go into panic mode every time newly recovered addicts go on an errand by themselves or spend an unusually long time in the bathroom.

It can be very helpful for families to be in some sort of therapy or support group during this period, to express their feelings and frustrations and share with others who are experiencing similar things.

It's important to understand that the feelings most family members have during this time are a normal reaction to the extreme stress caused by living with an addict during active addiction. Many families describe what they are going through as a kind of posttraumatic stress disorder, or PTSD. Thinking of the problem in that way can sometimes help families cope better with their own emotions and put less pressure on the recovering addict at a time when he or she is unlikely to be able to handle it.

Technically, the term "PTSD" describes the reaction of someone to a sudden event involving grievous bodily harm, not to the aftermath of a highly stressful living situation. Nevertheless, the symptoms can be remarkably similar. One family member of an addict joked that "I suffer from OTSD—*ongoing* traumatic stress disorder."

AFTERCARE PLANNING

Because recovering addicts need ongoing support, most detox facilities will help an addict with some sort of aftercare planning—which may include therapy, drug treatments, and attendance at support-group meetings.

The aftercare plan may include a stint at rehab. If so, the rehab facility will then usually help the addict with an aftercare plan for when the addict leaves that facility.

Following the aftercare plan can be crucial during this period, given that the addict's brain is still recovering and he or she is likely to be in a fragile state.

In addition to meetings and therapy, some aftercare plans include a recovery coach, someone who is not a therapist but is trained and available as needed to assist the addict in early recovery. Coaches may help recovering addicts find support-group meetings they will like, direct them to other types of resources, provide transportation, discuss issues in their life, arrange a sober companion for difficult periods when the addict will be alone, and otherwise offer support.

Recovery coaches can also provide periodic "check-ups" for people in longer-term recovery to address any issues they may be having.

Recently there has been a movement to certify recovery coaches as part of a new quasi-professional field. Coaches are not inexpensive, but they can be a valuable bridge for some people.

Sometimes an aftercare plan will include drug or alcohol testing, to make sure the addict is staying clean and sober and to catch any relapses before they spiral out of control. Regular or random testing can provide accountability to the recovering addict and can help prevent relapse. Family members can perform these tests themselves using relatively inexpensive over-the-counter test kits; they can also use a third-party sobriety-monitoring program. (See Chapter 20 for more information on drug testing.)

SOBER-LIVING HOMES

An important question for recovering addicts, especially young adults, is where they will live after detox or rehab. If they were previously living on their own, they can go back to their old home, but this might not always be advisable. Going home means being exposed again to all the same conditions, environments, and friends that the addict was used to when he or she was using. Being put back into the same environment can often weaken an addict's resolve and trigger relapse. Addicts who were living with their parents can go back to their parents' home, but this can cause the same problems. And some parents don't want the addict living at home, for the reasons given here or because they don't feel that they can provide as much support as the addict needs. In such cases, a sober-living home can be a good idea.

Sober-living homes are group homes for recovering addicts. They are different from rehabs in that they don't offer treatment. (Some people refer to sober-living homes as halfway houses, but this can be confusing because the term "halfway house" is more commonly used for residences for released convicts or people with different psychiatric issues.)

Sober-living residents can come and go as they please, but they are typically required to follow a number of rules. Generally, they must pay rent and help with chores around the house. They must be working, looking for work, or in school. They may have to attend regular meetings of house members. The most important rule is that they must stay clean and sober and not bring drugs or alcohol into the house. The house typically has a staff that keeps tabs on residents and enforces the rules.

Residents are often subject to random drug tests and to nightly curfews. They may also be required to go to Twelve-Step meetings or therapy (although the sober-living home will probably not itself provide the meetings or therapy). Violating the rules can lead to eviction. Residents can also be evicted if they fight or are unable to get along with other residents.

The rent is typically the same as for a modest apartment in the area, although there are now an increasing number of luxury sober-living homes that are more expensive and offer more amenities. Unlike renting an apartment, it's common for residents not to have to pay the last month's rent in advance, not to have to sign a year-long lease, and not to have to pay for utilities. There's no "standard" length of stay at a sober-living home; how long people stay depends on their unique situation and needs.

Some sober-living homes require new residents to have completed a rehab program, but not all do. Most will at least require a resident to have gone through a medical detox, although some will accept anyone who is currently clean and sober.

Some sober-living homes are single-sex, and some are coed. Coed facilities often forbid residents from having romantic relationships with other residents.

Not all residents are young adults. Older people may choose a sober-living home because they feel that they need a more structured environment, because they lost their previous home during active addiction, or because their spouse wants time apart from them.

Some sober-living homes are very strict; others are much looser. It's worth comparing them to see what works best in a specific circumstance. For some recovering addicts, an overly strict environment can make them feel anxious and stressed and more likely to want to use, while others are more likely to relapse in a less controlled environment.

It's also worth considering a sober-living home that is in a different geographic setting. Getting completely away from the area can help an addict avoid environments associated with substance use and contribute to the sense of "starting a new life."

What Causes Relapse?

"Relapse" means that an addict in recovery goes back to using. Relapse can happen at any time. It's particularly common in the first year of recovery, and especially in the first few weeks and months, because addicts' brains are still healing from the biochemical changes wrought by the disease, and they are only just beginning to learn how to construct a new life based on something other than substance abuse. However, addiction is a lifelong chronic illness, and relapse can still occur even after many years of being clean and sober.

The exact causes of relapse are different for each person, and there's seldom one specific prompt; it's most often a combination of a variety of factors. However, scientists believe that the general *types* of things that can cause relapse are fairly common across individuals.

RELAPSE TRIGGERS

Things that are likely to prompt relapse are often referred to as "triggers" or "cues." In general, there are three types of relapse triggers: stress, exposure to the substance of choice, and cues in the environment.

Stress

A very large number of addicts use substances to self-medicate against stress and anxiety. Thus, stress is a trigger because it causes the recovering addict to want to reach for the antidote that has seemingly worked so well in the past. Also, particularly in early recovery, the addict is working very hard to cope with the circumstances of life while maintaining the resolve not to go back to using. Stress makes it harder to cope with life and thus makes it harder to maintain one's resolve.

Exposure to the Substance

Being exposed to the addict's drug of choice—for instance, a recovering alcoholic going into a bar—can be a powerful trigger. Exposure to a substance can also include exposure to related items, such as drug paraphernalia or empty beer bottles.

This seems rather obvious, since exposure to a drug causes temptation. But there's more to it than that. Studies have shown that even seeing a picture of something associated with drug use—such as a syringe or a mound of white powder—can cause a sudden release of dopamine in the nucleus accumbens, or pleasure center, of an addict's brain. In effect, the exposure causes a miniature high similar to that of taking the drug itself. This can restart the brain's biochemical addiction process. The resulting cravings can be very difficult to overcome, especially if the prefrontal cortex or rational decision-making part of the brain is still "under repair."

One of the reasons the cravings may be hard to overcome is that the whole process can work subconsciously. For instance, one remarkable study found that images relating to cocaine use could trigger a dopamine reaction in the brain even though addicts were exposed to them for only 33 thousandths of a second—far too quickly for them to register consciously.

Many alcoholics have described relapse as something that seemed to happen to them suddenly, without warning, and without their remembering making a conscious decision to imbibe. In Alcoholics Anonymous parlance, they were "struck drunk." Scientifically speaking, they may have been overwhelmed by an unconscious dopamine process.

Environmental Cues

The term "environmental cues" refers to exposure, not to a substance itself, but to other things that addicts mentally associate with their prior use. It might refer to a room where they got high, a particular liquor store, a street corner where they bought drugs, friends they used to spend time with while using, certain types of music, or any number of other things.

In the famous "Pavlov's dog" experiment, Dr. Ivan Pavlov activated a metronome whenever he gave a dog food. He showed that the dog would eventually associate the two and start to salivate whenever it heard the metronome, even if food wasn't present. In much the same way, addicts associate their substance of choice with the things that were present when they used it. Simply being around those things can trigger a dopamine reaction in the brain that can make it much harder not to fall into old patterns.

RELAPSE IS A PROCESS

Despite the fact that many people describe being "struck drunk," most professionals believe that relapse is a process. Just as addiction doesn't happen overnight, relapse doesn't either; it's the result of a long series of choices that ultimately culminate in an addict "suddenly" relapsing.

For instance, a recovering alcoholic might be "struck drunk" after going into a bar, but why was he in a bar in the first place? Looking backward, you might find that he was experiencing a great deal of stress in his life. This caused him to miss meetings or therapy sessions, so he didn't get the support he needed. Exposure to environmental cues might have further weakened his resolve, and he began thinking wistfully about the "good times" when he was drinking. (Addicts often experience a kind of selective amnesia or "euphoric recall" where they remember the pleasant things about substance abuse and forget all the horrible things.) When someone invited him to a bar, he didn't have the resolve to say no, or he mistakenly believed that he could handle it. The relapse appeared sudden, but it was in fact the last step in a long chain of decisions and experiences.

Relapse isn't *solely* a function of triggers. The underlying chemical process in the brain is the real culprit, and the triggers are just a spark that's capable of starting a fire. It's possible to relapse without any exposure to triggers at all, but triggers certainly do not help.

HOW COMMON IS RELAPSE?

It's difficult for scientists to come up with precise statistics on relapse rates. This is true for a number of reasons, such as:

- It's impractical to follow addicts for the rest of their lives, so a study must have an arbitrary cutoff point. If a survey looks at how frequently addicts relapse within the first year, for instance, it will miss everyone who relapses after that . . . and it will be hard to compare that study to others that followed addicts for more or less time.
- What counts as a relapse? If someone "slips up" and has a couple drinks at a party, but immediately realizes the mistake and doesn't do it again, does that count?
- If someone resolves to give up drug use but starts using again after a very brief period, is that a relapse, or was the person never really clean to begin with?
- Some people are chronic relapsers and go back to using a dozen times or more. These people tend to skew any survey results.

In general, the difficulty of determining relapse rates is similar to the difficulty of calculating a "success rate" for Alcoholics Anonymous (see Chapter 29).

One of the most commonly cited statistics, and one mentioned by the U.S. National Institute on Drug Abuse, is that relapse rates range from 40 to 60 percent. This is comparable to relapse rates for people who receive treatment for other chronic conditions such as diabetes, heart disease, and asthma.

Certain groups may be more at risk. Some studies suggest that relapse rates are higher for women than for men; others suggest that they're higher for opioid addicts than for alcoholics. People who have co-occurring psychological disorders are also at greater risk for relapse. (However, every addict is different, and general statistics cannot predict how well a given person is likely to fare in recovery.)

One thing that studies consistently tend to show is that the longer people stay clean and sober, the more likely it is that they will continue to do so. A person who has five years of sobriety is much less likely to go back to drinking than a person who has been sober for only six months.

RELAPSE CAN BE DANGEROUS

Although it might seem like it to family members at the time, relapse is not necessarily the end of the world. Many addicts relapse once or even multiple times before achieving long-term recovery. Some addicts report that relapse was a valuable learning experience for them, showing them where their vulnerabilities were and where they needed to focus more attention.

However, it's also true that relapse can be dangerous. An addict who relapses doesn't just start over at the beginning and go through the whole long process of becoming addicted all over again. The addiction process causes permanent changes in the way the brain functions. As a result, addicts who go back to using after a long period of sobriety tend to pick up exactly where they left off. However sick they were at the time they quit, they tend to go back to that point as soon as they start using again. That makes relapse hard to recover from—addicts who relapse for a month don't just have to recover from a month of drinking or taking drugs; they have to recover all over again from the years of drinking or taking drugs that occurred before that.

Something that can make relapse especially dangerous is that, while addicts who relapse tend to go right back to where they were in terms of brain functioning, their body's tolerance level has changed. Thus, when they go back to using, they are likely to begin at the same level of consumption as where they left off—but their body might no longer be able to handle it. For instance, alcoholics who previously drank several bottles of wine a day might go back to the same habit, but they might become extremely sick because their body is no longer used to that level of alcohol.

More dangerously, a heroin addict who relapses is at greater risk of overdose. Heroin overdose occurs because excessive amounts of the drug enter the brainstem and depress the body's respiratory functions, causing the person to stop breathing. When a person is regularly using heroin, the brainstem adapts, meaning that the person can gradually take higher and higher doses of the drug and not have a respiratory failure. When the person goes without the drug for a while, however, the brainstem reverts to normal. As a result, if the person relapses and suddenly starts taking the same dose that he or she was used to in the past, the brainstem may be overwhelmed, and death can result.

This is why you hear so many stories of celebrities and others overdosing on heroin immediately after a relapse. Their brain's pleasure center was in one place, but their brainstem was in another. This is why it's critical for anyone living with an opioid addict to keep Narcan on hand to reverse an overdose—even if the addict is in recovery. (See Chapter 20 for more information on Narcan.)

35

How to Prevent Relapse

There are a number of things that addicts and their families can do to lessen the chance of relapse, ranging from commonsense practices to classes and techniques created by behavioral psychologists.

As discussed in the last chapter, relapse is most often precipitated by triggers—including stress, exposure to a substance, and environmental cues. Thus, a good commonsense practice is to avoid these triggers as much as possible.

DEALING WITH STRESS

In the case of stress, of course, avoiding it is easier said than done. But routines such as getting enough sleep, eating well, and regular exercise can help. That's why these habits are generally promoted in residential rehab programs.

Exercise

Exercise is particularly valuable. You may have heard that aerobic exercise produces endorphins, which for years were associated with the so-called "runner's high." Endorphins are a natural painkiller, structurally similar to morphine but not addictive. But while exercise increases the number of endorphins in the blood, there's little evidence that it increases the number of endorphins in the brain, so it might not be responsible for as many of the happy feelings that come from exercise as was first thought.

What exercise does do in the brain, however, is to increase the level of several other neurotransmitters, including serotonin, norepinephrine, and anandamide. These neurotransmitters can reduce depression and stress. What's more, many scientists believe that producing them through exercise actually trains the brain to respond more effectively to stress. In effect, exercise gives the body practice in responding to stressful situations and streamlines the communication system between the parts of the brain that are involved in stress response. The brains of people who don't exercise are simply not as efficient at producing the chemicals that help them cope with anxiety and depression, and so they are more likely to be overwhelmed by negative feelings.

Yoga

As part of helping with stress reduction, some residential rehab programs offer classes in yoga and meditation. (And some include other techniques such as acupuncture, art therapy, and pet visits.) Yoga and meditation can obviously be practiced outside rehab, and many recovering addicts find them helpful in maintaining equanimity in the face of stress.

Yoga is a complex Indian spiritual tradition. When most people in the West talk about yoga, they are referring to a particular branch of yoga called *hatha* yoga, which includes a collection of physical postures and practices that can be engaged in without reference to any larger spiritual ideal. Like aerobic exercise, these postures and practices have been shown to reduce anxiety and depression and help the brain learn how to respond more effectively to stress.

Meditation

Meditation typically involves sitting quietly and focusing the brain on a particular sound, called a mantra, or on one's body or breathing. A common goal is to induce a state of consciousness where one is aware of one's thoughts but able to detach oneself from them—to experience them as an observer rather than identifying with them. One is aware that the thought arose but simply accepts it and lets it go.

Regular meditation can train the brain to do much the same thing in daily life—to acknowledge thoughts that are stressful, anxious, or depressed, but not to get "stuck" in them, and to see them as a passing condition or one possible viewpoint rather than the only truth. This can help a person cope with stress and find effective solutions to daily problems rather than simply feeling anxious and worried about them.

Meditation is a part of many religious traditions, but (as with yoga) the practice can be separated from the religious background. Interestingly, meditation is specifically mentioned in the eleventh of the Twelve Steps of Alcoholics Anonymous, although the sense of the term as it is used there is probably closer to contemplation in general than to a particular mind-training technique.

AVOIDING THE SUBSTANCE

As for the second type of trigger, exposure to the substance, this would seem to be a lot easier to avoid than stress. Obviously, a recovering heroin addict should avoid being around heroin, and a gambling addict should stay away from a casino. But avoiding one's drug of choice can be a lot more difficult in the case of alcoholics because alcohol is so ubiquitous in our culture.

Family members can help here in a number of ways. One is to rid the addict's home of any alcohol. (This can involve even nonobvious alcohol, such as cooking sherry, and switching to an alcohol-free mouthwash.) Family members can also swear off drinking themselves when they are around the addict. Sometimes a recovering addict will feel guilty about depriving family members of the pleasure and encourage them to have a drink at a restaurant, saying, "Go ahead; I don't mind." However, whatever addicts may say, refraining from drinking alcohol around them is very respectful and always a good idea.

Some recovering alcoholics want to try drinking nonalcoholic beer or wine. In general, most professionals think this is not a good idea. For one thing, "nonalcoholic" beers and wines actually do contain small amounts of alcohol. Also, they bring the addict's attention back to drinking alcohol—and even though it might not literally be drinking alcohol, it can amount to a trigger. (A joke among some AA members is "Nonalcoholic beer is fine—for nonalcoholics.")

Avoiding exposure to alcohol can be especially difficult on certain occasions, such as holidays, parties, and weddings. Extended family who show up for holidays might not know about the addict's condition or might not realize that drinking around the person is a bad idea. At parties and weddings, there's really no effective way to prevent exposure to alcohol (and at some parties, illegal drugs). A recovering addict can choose not to go to family holiday gatherings or weddings, but doing so can create a number of other problems and can sometimes backfire by increasing the addict's stress level.

Also, some addicts in early recovery are overconfident about their abilities and will reassure everyone that going to a party is not going to create a problem. That might be true, but it also might not be.

When exposure to alcohol is unavoidable, it can be a good idea for family members to talk openly with the addict ahead of time and come up with a strategy. For instance, family members might take turns spending time with the addict at the event or otherwise keeping an eye on the person to make sure everything is okay. The family might agree on a "safe word" that the addict can use to communicate to a family member that he or she is feeling shaky. The family can then execute a prearranged plan to remove the addict at least temporarily from the gathering, using an excuse that everyone has agreed on in advance.

In many areas, Alcoholics Anonymous groups hold "alcathons"— all-day drop-in meetings on difficult holidays such as Christmas and New Year's Eve. (AA members sometimes joke that they refer to New Year's Eve as "amateur night.")

AVOIDING ENVIRONMENTAL CUES

As for the third type of trigger, environmental cues, this is complicated and highly specific to the addict's experience. Some addicts who associate using substances with a particular room in their home will choose to move, or redecorate, or spend time away at a sober-living home. Many will try to avoid contact with former friends whom they associate with using. Some people—especially young adults—will relocate to a different part of the country to achieve a fresh start.

Of course, avoiding environmental cues doesn't necessarily require such a radical change. It can often involve making much smaller and subtler alterations in one's life. It all depends on the addict's own unique experience.

AVOIDING CROSS-ADDICTIONS

Most addicts have a particular drug of choice, but people who are susceptible to becoming addicted to one thing are often at greater risk of becoming addicted to another. As a result, it's often a good idea for people in recovery to avoid contact not only with the substance to which they were addicted, but also with other substances that are addictive in nature.

Many people say that they have given up heroin and "only" smoke marijuana, or have kicked their cocaine habit but still like to go out drinking. Maybe this works, but a lot of professionals believe that this type of behavior is a red flag. For one thing, it shows some vulnerability in the person's resolve to fully engage in recovery—many addicts will simply substitute one substance for another when they're early in the process and still feeling ambivalent about abstinence. For another, it creates the risk of developing a cross-addiction to the other substance.

The good news is that researchers have found that a person who succeeds in kicking one substance abuse habit is more likely to be able to kick another.

Families can be very supportive in early recovery by ridding a house of alcohol and not drinking around a recovering addict, even if the addict is recovering from something other than alcoholism.

Cigarettes

The issue of cross-addiction comes up frequently when people who are recovering from an alcohol or drug addiction either take up or continue smoking cigarettes. After all, nicotine is an addictive substance, and while it doesn't tend to cause the devastating behavioral changes associated with alcoholism or heroin addiction, it can certainly be deadly in the long term.

The Alcoholics Anonymous Big Book, which dates from the 1930s, encourages families not to worry about tobacco use and instead to focus on the problem of alcoholism. Of course, the book was published long before the full health effects of tobacco were widely known.

Smoking among alcoholics is common. A study conducted in 1998 found that as many as 90 percent of alcoholics were smokers, and a 2008 survey found that 57 percent of recovering alcoholics who participated in AA smoked.

Many professionals who treat alcoholism believe that smoking is a lesser issue and that it should be addressed later, once the person's alcohol use is under control. On the other hand, there's research suggesting that treating people for alcoholism and nicotine addiction at the same time is beneficial because addressing one problem actually makes it easier to address the other. There's also early research suggesting that people who successfully quit smoking during early recovery feel less depressed and are less likely to relapse.

RELAPSE PREVENTION THERAPY

One of the earliest attempts by professionals to create a formal strategy for avoiding relapse was relapse prevention therapy, or RPT. In recent years a large number of scientific studies have demonstrated the effectiveness of this approach.

RPT focuses particularly on high-risk situations—those where a recovering addict is especially likely to begin using again. A primary goal of the therapy is to work with addicts to identify such situations and to equip them with coping skills to resist the resulting temptation.

RPT believes that the simple process of identifying these situations is helpful in itself because it allows addicts to realize where their weak points are and where they need to be most careful. Beyond that, RPT therapists work with addicts to develop effective responses—for example, planning in advance what to say if someone offers them a drink at a party. The therapist might also role-play the situation, so addicts can practice responding and be prepared to cope with the scenario confidently.

RPT also encourages thinking about ways to avoid high-risk situations altogether.

Another element of RPT is teaching the addict that avoiding relapse is not a matter of sheer willpower; it's a set of new skills to be mastered. The idea is that addicts will feel empowered because they can actually do something positive, as opposed to simply trying to resist something negative. RPT also teaches the addict to focus on small, achievable tasks (such as getting through a particular high-risk situation) rather than larger and more daunting goals (such as a lifetime of abstinence). In this way, it's similar to the popular saying in Alcoholics Anonymous, "One day at a time."

Reframing

Yet another focus of RPT is cognitive restructuring or "reframing." This means using education and reminders to change the way the addict thinks about things. For example, many recovering alcoholics have positive memories of how alcohol made them feel or how it helped them deal with awkwardness in social situations. An RPT therapist can help them supplement their memories of positive feelings with all the now-forgotten memories of very negative things they experienced while engaged in heavy drinking.

The therapist can also tell them about scientific research showing that the perceived social benefits of alcohol are either nonexistent or the result, not of alcohol itself, but of the drinker's own expectations about it. In other words, alcohol doesn't actually make people more effective socially; it merely functions as a placebo.

Urge Surfing

Another reframing technique teaches the addict that urges and cravings don't reflect a genuine desire to drink or use drugs but are a normal conditioned physiological response to an external stimulus. The response is much like that of Pavlov's dog, who automatically started salivating when he heard the metronome. Addicts are taught to detach themselves from the craving and to watch it as an observer.

In a technique called urge surfing, the addict is instructed to imagine the urge as a wave, or series of waves, and to experience them as building and crashing. The addict eventually learns that cravings don't actually build and build consistently until they become overwhelming; rather, they tend to dissipate fairly quickly if the addict doesn't act on them. The goal is to "surf" the crave waves and avoid being swept away by them.

OTHER THERAPY TECHNIQUES

Here's a look at some other therapy techniques that are used to help addicts avoid relapse.

Coping Skills Training

Coping skills training is a broad attempt to help the recovering addict deal better with life. The premise is that the addict in the past has relied on only one method (the substance of choice) for handling the demands of living. As a result, his or her general coping skills and effectiveness in dealing with life's requirements have been impaired. The more addicts can develop positive coping skills, the less likely they will be to fall back on their old method of substance abuse.

Technically, RPT is a subset of coping skills training that focuses on high-risk situations. Other elements of coping skills training include improving social skills in general, developing better communication habits, and learning to manage one's moods.

Mindfulness-Based Relapse Prevention

Mindfulness-based relapse prevention, or MBRP, combines RPT with meditation and other mindfulness-based stress-reduction techniques. The goal is to help recovering addicts accept cravings and temptations but mentally detach from them rather than immediately reaching for a "fix."

At least one scientific study has shown that MBRP is effective in reducing relapse rates.

Behavior Chain Analysis

Behavior chain analysis is a major component of cognitive-behavioral therapy (which is discussed in Chapter 26). The idea is to look at a specific problematic behavior and examine the situation that immediately preceded the behavior. The person then reflects on the thoughts, emotions, and sensations caused by the situation. The theory is that certain negative thoughts started a "chain" of negative emotions and reactions that ultimately led to the behavior.

By reflecting on these thoughts, the person can often come up with more positive and rational thoughts that are equally valid reactions to the same situation and that are less likely to lead to self-destructive responses. The person can then respond to similar situations in the future with more affirmative thoughts, more positive emotions, and more constructive behaviors.

Behavior chain analysis is useful in helping people in active addiction to identify what causes them to use substances, but it can also be helpful to recovering addicts in enabling them to identify relapse triggers and change the thought processes that make relapse more likely.

Contingency Management

Contingency management is a program that pays or otherwise rewards people for avoiding relapse. For instance, recovering addicts might receive a reward every time they pass a drug test, take medication as prescribed, or attend a scheduled therapy session. Rewards might include small vouchers that are redeemable for consumer goods. (Vouchers are generally used because, unlike cash, they can't be spent on alcohol or drugs.) Sometimes the reward is a chance to draw from a bowl for a larger prize. The person gets additional draws for each week of successfully completing the treatment requirements; a violation means the person must start over at the beginning.

In some programs, methadone users who pass drug tests for three months may be given one "take-home" dose per week, which is a reward because it means that the person doesn't have to travel to the clinic.

Paying people not to relapse may sound odd, but there are a number of studies showing that a system of small tangible rewards can improve results. As with RPT, it works on the principle that addicts fare better if they see relapse prevention as doing something positive rather than just avoiding something negative.

Contingency management is designed for addicts in early recovery programs, to help them through the crucial first few months. The goal is to wean them off the rewards system once they have developed other relapse-avoidance skills.

Despite the fact that research shows the benefits of contingency management, many institutions are reluctant to try it because they believe that it raises difficult ethical, tax, and oversight issues.

36

What to Do
If a Relapse Happens

There are two ways of thinking about relapse. You could call them the hard way and the soft way.

The hard way is that relapse is completely unacceptable. It amounts to a failure of treatment. The addict has fallen apart and is no longer in recovery; he or she is back at square one.

An example of the hard way might be the tradition of sobriety chips in Alcoholics Anonymous. Many AA members receive chips, similar to poker chips, to represent various sobriety milestones—one day, one month, 6 months, a year, and so on. The chips recognize accomplishment, but if a person relapses, he or she literally goes back to "square one" and must start all over again with the one-day chip. Any previous time sober doesn't count. This suggests that relapse undoes everything that went before. (While sobriety chips are very common in AA, the practice isn't officially recognized by the AA organization and many groups do not use them.)

The soft way of thinking about relapse recognizes that relapse is extremely common—in fact, a frequently cited statistic is that 40 to 60 percent of addicts relapse at some point. The soft way doesn't view relapse as a failure that undoes everything that came before; rather, it views it as a bump in the road that shows that more treatment is needed and where the addict's vulnerabilities are. In this view, relapse is a normal part of the recovery process.

There's no one right way to think about relapse. Both alternatives have their advantages.

The good thing about the hard way is that it can help a recovering addict avoid temptation. It adds weight to the scale on the side of not using. Addicts who think that a year or more of sobriety can be undone by a single mistake, and that they will have to go back to the beginning and start all over again (and receive another one-day chip), might be highly motivated to stay sober.

On the other hand, if a relapse does occur, the soft way might be the better approach to take when reacting to it. An addict who comes to view relapse as a personal failure rather than a normal part of the process might be more inclined to give up hope and not make an effort to get back to sobriety. He or she might be filled with feelings of worthlessness, self-blame, and anxiety, which can in turn trigger further relapsing.

There are scientific studies that back up this view. Researchers asked addicts who had relapsed about their attitudes toward the relapse and then compared the long-term results. What they found is that addicts who were filled with shame and viewed the relapse as a failure were more likely to go back to chronic substance abuse, whereas addicts who viewed the relapse as a transitional learning experience were more likely to experiment with alternative coping strategies and work their way back to being clean and sober.

For this reason, many professionals think that adopting an approach based on the soft way is preferable once a relapse has occurred. They encourage families not to inflict blame, anger, or guilt on the addict. They promote an attitude of "This is just something that shows us where we have more work to do. We'll come back from it and do even better."

Another problem with families adopting the hard way is that it might encourage an addict to hide the fact of a relapse and not tell the truth, which makes it more difficult to get help and support and may lead to a more serious relapse episode. One of the first things that families are often advised to say when an addict confesses to a relapse is "Thank you for being honest."

Of course, it's not always easy for families to be supportive once a relapse occurs. Family members may well be full of anger and resentment and feel that the addict has let them down and that all their hard work has been for nothing. Indeed, adopting the soft-way attitude can be a much harder thing for families than for addicts themselves.

RELAPSE VERSUS A "SLIP"

Some people draw a distinction between a slip—a very brief return to substance use—and a full-blown relapse where the person goes back to uncontrollable addictive behavior.

A slip might include having a couple drinks at a party, a single instance of drug use, or a single trip to a casino. In this view, one of the goals of relapse prevention is to stop a single or occasional slip from spiraling into a full-blown relapse.

One way to do this is with slip planning. Family members can assure the recovering addict that they understand that slips are possible and that the most important thing is for the addict to be honest about them should they occur. The addict needs to be reassured that slips will be met with understanding, rather than anger and blame, so that he or she will feel comfortable being honest. Next, the family (including the addict) should work out a plan for exactly what will happen in the event of a slip. Will the person go back to rehab, and if so, where? What other steps will be taken? This can be done in conjunction with a therapist or counselor.

The first goal of this type of planning is to eliminate the panic that so often sets in (on the part of both the addict and the family) when relapse occurs. Everyone knows what the plan is and how to react, so they can simply carry it out. The second goal is to encourage a quick intervention as soon as a slip happens, so as to keep a brief mistake from spiraling out of control.

Some people object to this kind of slip planning on the grounds that it normalizes slips in the addict's mind and makes the addict think that slipping is okay. That's a legitimate criticism, one based on the hard way of thinking about relapse. In the end, each family has to decide for itself what approach it is most comfortable with.

CHRONIC RELAPSE

While a large number of recovering addicts relapse once or twice, there are some who relapse over and over again. This is called chronic relapse.

Chronic relapsers tend to fall into two types. The first are addicts who generally want to get well—hence their continuing attempts at recovery each time they relapse—but who for whatever reason have enormous trouble getting over the initial hurdle of staying clean. These people often have especially strong post-acute withdrawal symptoms, and have great difficulty controlling their impulses long enough for the brain to heal and for the prefrontal cortex to return to more normal functioning.

Often these addicts seem to relapse on a timetable. For instance, they might be able to put together 60 days of sobriety, but that's when they fall apart. Although it's expensive, such addicts might be particularly suited to a longer residential (or at least outpatient) treatment period, such as 90 days, to help them get through the initial phase of withdrawal and healing. Some out-of-the-box thinking might help too. For instance, although people typically go to rehab immediately after detox, these addicts might benefit from delaying the start of rehab until shortly before the first 60 days are up.

The second type of chronic relapsers are people who have learned to "work the system." Unlike the first type, these are people who don't actually have much desire to get well. They are treatment-savvy, understand the "lingo" of addiction and recovery, and have learned to use the system to further their bad habits.

Such addicts can be highly manipulative and willing to exploit any tendency toward enabling on the part of family and friends. They often go into treatment simply because their money and options have temporarily run out, and detox or rehab gives them a place to stay and something to eat. They will say whatever the staff members want to hear, but once they get out, they go back to using—until the next time they need a place to "crash."

There's not a lot that can be done for such addicts, although a strict refusal by the family to engage in any type of enabling may help. Some professionals have suggested that this type of chronic relapser may benefit from extremely long residential treatment—say, nine months to a year to break their pattern of behavior—although this is obviously financially out of the question for most people.

Managing Addiction
as a Long-Term
Chronic Illness

There is no cure for addiction, or at least researchers haven't come close to finding one.

A true cure would mean that the addict's brain would no longer be in danger of creating a downward spiral induced by dopamine. An alcoholic could have a drink or two at a party and be fine. An opioid addict could be prescribed a painkiller as needed. A gambling addict could spend an hour at a casino and then leave without a further thought about it.

Unfortunately, a cure doesn't seem to be on even the distant horizon. In part, that's because we still understand so little about why some people are susceptible to addiction and others aren't. In part, too, it's because what we *do* know suggests that it's not just a simple medical phenomenon that could be attacked with a pill or a vaccine. It's a complex interplay of biological, genetic, psychological, and environmental factors that are unique to each individual.

That's not to say that some people haven't tried. From time to time, for instance, a few scientists have published results suggesting that alcoholics can be returned to a pattern of moderate drinking. But other researchers haven't been able to replicate the results, and long-term follow-up studies of the "moderate" drinkers have often shown that they weren't able to keep up the pattern for long without returning to addictive behavior.

In short, for the time being the only totally safe solution we have is complete abstinence from the addictive substance.

Thus, a good way to think of addiction is as a long-term chronic illness. It's similar to diabetes, in that we can't "fix" the pancreas, but people with diabetes can live a rich, full life as long as they watch what they eat and take insulin if needed.

With other chronic illnesses such as diabetes, heart disease, kidney disease, and so on, we tend to think of the life changes a person has to make as primarily physical. They involve diet, exercise, medication, and perhaps a procedure such as dialysis. But the truth is that coping with a chronic illness is also a psychological process. It's not easy to make wholesale changes to your diet, take up a regular exercise regimen, or limit your participation in activities you have always enjoyed (as most anyone who has tried it will tell you). Doing so usually involves a reorganization of how one thinks about life in general. Also, drugs and medical procedures often have their own psychological effects to which the person must learn to adapt, and simply accepting the fact that the rest of one's life will be significantly altered by an illness is in itself psychologically difficult.

Addiction is similar in this respect—and in fact with addiction the need for a psychological reorganization may be even more profound. After all, addiction specifically targets the brain, and one of its primary effects is altering the way the person makes judgments about what's most important in life. Managing addiction as a chronic illness doesn't just mean abstaining from substances; it means finding a new way of coping with all of life's challenges.

Looking back, many people in recovery say that the way they lived before they became addicts was less than ideal. Many say that they often experienced depression, loneliness, low self-esteem, or a generalized anxiety. Addiction "solved" this problem by taking away those feelings. Of course, it didn't really solve the problem at all; it made the addict's life much worse. But the fact that an addict has finally succeeded in stopping using a substance doesn't mean that the underlying feelings that the substance was medicating have gone away. The addict still has to learn to deal with those feelings and find a more constructive way of living.

An important distinction can be made between "abstinence" and "recovery." Some people can stop using, at least for a time, without making any underlying changes in their lives—AA calls these people dry drunks—but such individuals are liable to relapse because the underlying psychological makeup that was present when they first started using is still there. The best way to avoid relapse over time—to manage addiction as a long-term chronic illness—is to find a more successful way of handling the underlying conflicts and challenges in one's personality. This is, in the fullest sense, the meaning of "recovery."

Some people accomplish this through psychotherapy that analyzes childhood experiences and long-term psychological issues. Some people engage in deep soul searching about what landed them in trouble with addiction in the first place. Some people find the courage to make changes in their lives that they knew for a long time they should make but were afraid to tackle. Some people make an effort to give back, either by helping other addicts in support-group meetings or finding other ways to volunteer in the community.

There's no one right way to live recovery. The causes of the illness are unique to each person, and so are the solutions.

Families, too, have to go through recovery. The family was organized in one way before and during the addiction. As the addict gets well, the family has to adapt to the changes that he or she is going through. And this can require family members to experience considerable soul searching and psychological growth as well.

AA describes recovery as a spiritual awakening. Other people have other ways of talking about it. One thing we can say for sure, though, is that addiction is a tragedy, for both the addict and the family. Many people who experience a tragedy in their life take a long time to come back from it, but when they do come back, they usually do so having changed in some fundamental way. People who have weathered a tragedy successfully—who have understood and accepted loss at a deep level—often develop personality traits such as compassion, patience, thoughtfulness, gratitude, emotional insight, and inner peace. They will tell you that they profoundly wish the tragedy had never happened, but that the experience has left them better, stronger, and more truly loving people than they were before.

And until there's a cure, this is the best thing that we can hope for.

Resources

H ere are some additional resources for families in the United States and other English-speaking countries. Preference has been given to governmental and independent nonprofit organizations, but some for-profit resources have also been included. Programs, websites, and phone numbers are of course subject to change, but every effort has been made to keep this list as current as possible.

FINDING TREATMENT PROGRAMS

Be careful! Many apparently official "helplines" and online directories are in fact run by for-profit treatment centers, and their main goal is to persuade you to use their services rather than to provide unbiased information and advice. If you find a directory of treatment programs online, be sure to click on the "About Us" link or otherwise research the organization that operates the directory. If a website is vague or unclear about the organization that operates it, that's a red flag. Also, note that directories run by for-profit companies in the United States typically have ".com" at the end of their web address, whereas those run by nonprofits usually end in ".org" and those run by government agencies usually end in ".gov."

In the United States

A list of addiction treatment programs (by ZIP code) is available on the U.S. Substance Abuse and Mental Health Services Administration website at *www. findtreatment.samhsa.gov.*

Helplines that provide referrals to local treatment facilities, support groups, and community-based organizations as well as additional information are operated by:

- The U.S. Substance Abuse and Mental Health Services Administration, at (800) 662-4357.
- The Addiction Policy Forum, at (833) 301-4357.

A list of alcoholism treatment programs (by ZIP code) is available on the website of the National Institute on Alcohol Abuse and Alcoholism at *www.alcohol treatment.niaaa.nih.gov/how-to-find-alcohol-treatment/find-alcohol-treatment-programs*.

A list of medication-assisted opioid treatment programs (by state) is available on the U.S. Substance Abuse and Mental Health Services Administration website at *https://dpt2.samhsa.gov/treatment*.

A list of doctors authorized to provide buprenorphine treatment (by ZIP code) can be found on the U.S. Substance Abuse and Mental Health Services Administration website at *www.samhsa.gov/medication-assisted-treatment/physician-program-data/treatment-physician-locator*.

A list of Vivitrol providers (by ZIP code) can be found at *www.vivitrol.com/find-a-treatment-provider*.

Directories of physicians who specialize in addiction treatment can be found on the following websites:

- The American Society of Addiction Medicine, at *http://asam.ps.membersuite.com/directory/SearchDirectory_Criteria.aspx*.
- The American Board of Addiction Medicine, at *www.abam.net/find-a-doctor*.
- The American Academy of Addiction Psychiatry, at *www.aaap.org/?page_id=658?sid=658*.
- The National Association of Addiction Treatment Providers, at *www.naatp.org/resources/addiction-industry-directory*.

A directory of psychologists who specialize in addiction can be found on the website of the American Psychological Association. Go to *http://locator.apa.org*, enter your ZIP code or city and state, and enter "addiction" as a specialty. The results page will tell you whether nearby psychologists are accepting new patients and what types of insurance they accept.

A directory of therapists who specialize in cognitive-behavioral therapy can be found on the website of the National Association of Cognitive-Behavioral Therapists at *www.nacbt.org/find-a-therapist*.

A directory of psychiatrists who specialize in teenagers can be found on the website of the American Academy of Child & Adolescent Psychiatry at *www.aacap.org/AACAP/Families_and_Youth/Resources/CAP_Finder.aspx*.

You can search for accredited rehab facilities on the website of the Commission on Accreditation of Rehabilitation Facilities, which certifies rehabs. The address is *www.carf.org/providerSearch.aspx*. (Note that CARF certifies all sorts of rehab facilities, not just those for addiction, but the "Advanced Search" option lets you narrow your search to opioid abuse, alcoholism, etc.)

People who can't afford private addiction treatment can often get help from a state-funded rehab program. A good way to find out what state-funded programs are available is to contact the state agency in charge of substance-abuse services. Detailed contact information for every state agency can be found at *www.samhsa.gov/sites/default/files/ssadirectory.pdf*. The U.S. Substance Abuse and Mental Health Services Administration helpline (see previous page) can also refer you to state-funded treatment programs and to facilities that charge on a sliding-fee scale or accept Medicare or Medicaid. The number is (800) 662-4357.

A book that contains descriptive reports of experiences in many different types of rehabs is Anne M. Fletcher, *Inside Rehab* (Penguin Books, 2013).

Outside the United States

Canada

Links to government-provided addiction services by province can be found at *www.canadiandrugrehabcentres.com/cgi-bin/government-drug-programs.cgi.*

A government-funded directory of programs in Ontario can be found at *www. connexontario.ca/Search/AdvancedSearch.*

A privately run but comprehensive list of programs by province can be found at *www.drugrehab.ca.*

A directory of government-funded programs for First Nations and Inuit peoples can be found at *www.canada.ca/en/indigenous-services-canada/services/ addictions-treatment-first-nations-inuit.html.*

United Kingdom

The NHS offers a directory of addiction services by location at *www.nhs.uk/ Service-Search/Drug%20treatment%20services/LocationSearch/340.*

Public Health England offers a rehab directory at *www.rehab-online.org.uk.*

A directory of treatment services in Scotland can be found at *www.scottish drugservices.com.*

Ireland

A searchable directory of addiction services can be found at *www.services. drugs.ie.*

A list of addiction services provided by the Health Service Executive is available at *www.hse.ie/eng/services/list/5/addiction.*

An alcoholism helpline run by the Health Service Executive can be contacted at 1800 459 459.

Australia

A national alcohol and drug hotline run by the Australian government can direct you to local services. The number is 1800 250 015.

A directory of Queensland treatment providers can be found at *www.qnada. org.au/service-finder/#.*

Another government-supported site that lets you search for local resources is *www.adin.com.au.*

New Zealand

A national alcohol and drug helpline can be contacted at 0800 787 797.

A list of additional resources provided by the Mental Health Education

& Resource Centre is available at *www.mherc.org.nz/directory/alcohol-drug-other-addiction-services.*

GETTING INSURANCE COVERAGE

In the United States

An interactive website that explains parity laws for mental and physical health insurance coverage and how they apply to addiction is operated by the U.S. Department of Health and Human Services. The address is *www.hhs.gov/programs/topic-sites/mental-health-parity/mental-health-and-addiction-insurance-help/index.html.*

If you have no insurance or are underinsured, the U.S. Substance Abuse and Mental Health Services Administration helpline can refer you to state-funded treatment programs and to facilities that charge on a sliding-fee scale or accept Medicare or Medicaid. The number is (800) 662-4357.

Another website that explains insurance coverage for addiction (albeit one run by a private rehab referral service) is *www.drugrehab.org/paying-for-drug-rehab-insurance-coverage.*

Australia

A useful website for understanding addiction insurance coverage (albeit one run by a private company) is *www.finder.com.au/health-insurance-for-drug-and-alcohol-treatments.*

SUPPORT GROUPS FOR ADDICTS

Twelve-Step Groups

Alcoholics Anonymous is the oldest and largest Twelve-Step group and has meetings in more than 90 countries.

- Main website: *www.aa.org.*
- To find meetings in the United States and Canada: *www.aa.org/pages/en_US/find-aa-resources.*
- To find meetings in other countries: *www.aa.org/pages/en_US/find-aa-resources/world/1.*
- To find online meetings: *www.aa-intergroup.org/directory.php.*

Narcotics Anonymous is a Twelve-Step group for drug addicts with meetings in more than 90 countries.

- Main website: *www.na.org.*
- To find meetings: *www.na.org/meetingsearch.*

Marijuana Anonymous offers meetings in the United States and nine other countries including Canada, the United Kingdom, Ireland, Australia, and New Zealand.

- Main website: *www.marijuana-anonymous.org.*
- To find meetings: *www.marijuana-anonymous.org/find-a-meeting.*

Cocaine Anonymous offers meetings in the United States and 24 other countries including Canada, the United Kingdom, Ireland, Australia, and New Zealand.

- Main website: *www.ca.org.*
- To find meetings: *www.ca.org/meetings.*
- To find online meetings: *www.ca-online.org/meetings.*

Heroin Anonymous offers meetings in the United States, Canada, the United Kingdom, and South Africa.

- Main website: *www.heroinanonymous.org.*
- To find meetings: *www.heroinanonymous.org/meetings.*

Crystal Meth Anonymous offers meetings in the United States and seven other countries including Canada, the United Kingdom, and Australia.

- Main website: *www.crystalmeth.org.*
- To find meetings: *www.crystalmeth.org/cma-meetings/cma-meetings-directory. html.*

Gamblers Anonymous offers meetings in the United States and almost 60 other countries including Canada, the United Kingdom, Ireland, Australia, and New Zealand.

- Main website: *www.gamblersanonymous.org.*
- To find meetings in the United States: *www.gamblersanonymous.org/ga/locations.*
- To find meetings in other countries: *www.gamblersanonymous.org/ga/ addresses.*

Overeaters Anonymous offers meetings in the United States and more than 80 other countries including Canada, the United Kingdom, Ireland, Australia, and New Zealand.

- Main website: *www.oa.org.*
- To find meetings: *www.oa.org/find-a-meeting/?type=0.*
- To find online meetings: *www.oa.org/find-a-meeting/?type=1.*

Food Addicts in Recovery Anonymous offers meetings in 10 countries including the United States, Canada, the United Kingdom, Australia, and New Zealand.

- Main website: *www.foodaddicts.org.*
- To find meetings: *www.foodaddicts.org/find-meeting.*

Spenders Anonymous offers meetings in about seven U.S. states as well as one in New Zealand.

- Main website: *www.spenders.org.*
- To find meetings: *www.spenders.org/list.html.*

Sex Addicts Anonymous offers meetings in the United States as well as Skype meetings in several languages.

- Main website: *www.saa-recovery.org.*
- To find meetings: *www.saa-recovery.org/meetings.*

Dual Recovery Anonymous is for people with an addiction and a separate emotional or psychiatric illness. It holds meetings in the United States, Canada, Australia, and New Zealand.

- Main website: *www.draonline.org.*
- To find meetings: *www.draonline.org/meetings.html.*

Secular AA offers online AA-type meetings without religious content. See *http://secularaa.org/on-line-meetings.*

Celebrate Recovery is a Christ-centered Twelve-Step program that offers meetings in the United States.

- Main website: *www.celebraterecovery.com.*
- To find meetings: *https://locator.crgroups.info.*

Online-only meetings are offered by a group called In The Rooms, at *www.intherooms.com.*

Other Groups

SMART Recovery is a nonreligious group that uses behavioral principles and addresses a wide variety of addiction issues. It offers meetings in the United States, Canada, the United Kingdom, and Australia.

- Main website: *www.smartrecovery.org.*
- To find meetings in the United States and Canada: *www.smartrecoverytest.org/local.*
- To find meetings in the United Kingdom: *www.smartrecovery.org.uk.*
- To find meetings in Australia: *www.smartrecoveryaustralia.com.au/find-meetings.*
- To find online meetings: *www.smartrecovery.org/community/calendar.php.*

Women for Sobriety is a female-only group for alcoholics and drug users. It offers meetings in the United States and Canada.

- Main website: *www.womenforsobriety.org.*
- To find meetings: *www.womenforsobriety.org/meetings.*

Secular Organizations for Sobriety addresses alcoholism, drug addiction, and overeating. It offers meetings in the United States and some other countries.

- Main website: *www.sossobriety.org.*
- To find meetings: *www.sossobriety.org/find-a-meeting.*

LifeRing Secular Recovery addresses alcoholism and drug addiction. It offers meetings in the United States, Canada, the United Kingdom, and Ireland.

- Main website: *www.lifering.org.*
- To find meetings: *www.lifering.org/find-a-lifering-meeting.*
- To find online meetings: *www.lifering.org/meeting-menu/online-meetings-chat-room/schedule-meeting-links/.*

Moderation Management is a group designed to reduce harm from drinking rather than promoting strict abstinence. It offers meetings in about 15 U.S. states and a few other countries.

- Main website: *www.moderation.org.*
- To find meetings: *www.moderation.org/meetings.*

SUPPORT GROUPS FOR FAMILIES

Twelve-Step Groups

Al-Anon is the largest support group for families of alcoholics and is based on Twelve-Step principles.

- Main website: *www.al-anon.org.*
- To find meetings in the United States: *www.al-anon.org/al-anon-meetings/find-an-al-anon-meeting.*
- To find meetings outside the United States: *www.al-anon.org/al-anon-meetings/worldwide-al-anon-contacts.*
- To find online meetings: *www.al-anon.org/al-anon-meetings/electronic-meetings.*

Alateen is a division of Al-Anon just for teenagers.

- Main website: *www.al-anon.org/for-members/group-resources/alateen.*
- To find meetings in the United States: *www.al-anon.org/al-anon-meetings/find-an-alateen-meeting.*
- To find meetings outside the United States: *www.al-anon.org/al-anon-meetings/worldwide-al-anon-contacts.*

Nar-Anon is similar to Al-Anon but is for families of drug addicts.

- Main website: *www.nar-anon.org.*

- To find meetings: *www.nar-anon.org/find-a-meeting.*

Narateen is a division of Nar-Anon just for teenagers.

- Main website: *www.nar-anon.org/narateen.*
- To find meetings: *www.nar-anon.org/find-a-meeting.*

Families Anonymous is another Twelve-Step group for families.

- Main website: *www.familiesanonymous.org.*
- To find meetings: *www.familiesanonymous.org/index.php?route=information/ information&information_id=21.*
- To find online meetings: *www.familiesanonymous.org/index. php?route=information/information&information_id=32.*

Gam-Anon is a Twelve-Step group for families of gambling addicts. It holds meetings in the United States and 10 other countries, including Canada, the United Kingdom, Australia, and New Zealand.

- Main website: *www.gam-anon.org.*
- To find meetings: *www.gam-anon.org/meeting-directory.*

Adult Children of Alcoholics is a Twelve-Step group that welcomes children of alcoholics, drug addicts, and dysfunctional families in general.

- Main website: *www.adultchildren.org.*
- To find meetings: *www.adultchildren.org/meeting-search.*

Co-Dependents Anonymous is a Twelve-Step group for people who may be experiencing codependency.

- Main website: *www.coda.org.*
- To find meetings in the United States: *http://locator.coda.org/index. cfm?page=usMeetings.cfm.*
- To find meetings in other countries: *http://locator.coda.org/index. cfm?page=intlMeetings.cfm.*
- To find online meetings: *http://locator.coda.org/index. cfm?page=onlineMeetings.cfm.*

Other Groups in the United States and Canada

A **searchable directory** of local meetings of a wide variety of family support groups in the United States can be found at *www.supportgroupproject.org.*

A **helpline that provides support for families** is offered by the Addiction Policy Forum at (833) 301-4357.

SMART Recovery Family & Friends is a support group for families that uses behavioral principles.

- Main website: *www.smartrecovery.org/family.*

- To find meetings: *www.smartrecoverytest.org/local.*
- To find online meetings: *www.smartrecovery.org/community/calendar.php.*

Parents of Addicted Loved Ones operates a number of meetings in Arizona, Indiana, and Kentucky, as well as at least one meeting in about 12 other U.S. states.

- Main website: *www.palgroup.org.*
- To find meetings: *www.palgroup.org/find-a-meeting.*

The National Alliance on Mental Illness offers support groups in the United States for family members of people suffering from mental illness in general.

- To find programs: *www.nami.org/Find-Support/NAMI-Programs.*

Because I Love You (BILY) offers support groups in the United States and Canada for parents of children (including adult children) who have behavioral problems, including drug and alcohol abuse.

- Main website: *www.bily.org.*
- To find meetings: *www.bily.org/get-help/meeting-locations.*

Shatterproof Family Support Programs are led by clinicians and trained coaches.

- Main website: *www.shatterproof.org/family.*
- For more information, contact (800) 597-2557 or info@shatterproof.org.

Learn to Cope offers meetings for families of drug addicts in Massachusetts.

- Main website: *www.learn2cope.org.*
- To find meetings: *www.learn2cope.org/meetings.*

Grief Recovery After a Substance Passing (GRASP) is a support group in the United States and Canada for family members who have lost a loved one due to addiction.

- Main website: *www.grasphelp.org.*
- To find meetings: *www.grasphelp.org/community/meetings.*

Other Groups Outside the United States and Canada

SMART Recovery Family & Friends (see previous page) is a support group for families that uses behavioral principles. It offers meetings in the United Kingdom, Ireland, and Australia as well as in the United States and Canada.

- Main website: *www.smartrecovery.org/family.*
- To find meetings: *www.smartrecoverytest.org/local.*
- To find online meetings: *www.smartrecovery.org/community/calendar.php.*

United Kingdom

Adfam offers more than 500 support groups for families. To find meetings: *www.adfam.org.uk/families/find_a_local_support_group.*

Ireland

The National Family Support Network offers family support groups. To find meetings: *www.fsn.ie/directory-of-groups.*

The Rise Foundation offers family educational programs and group therapy. See *www.therisefoundation.ie/family-programmes-and-1-1-counselling-service.html.*

Australia

Family Drug Support Australia offers many family support groups. To find meetings: *www.fds.org.au/meetings-and-events/family-support-meetings.*

NARCAN/NALOXONE

Detailed information on Narcan is available on the website of the National Institute on Drug Abuse at *www.drugabuse.gov/related-topics/opioid-overdose-reversal-naloxone-narcan-evzio,* and on the website of the Addiction Policy Forum at *www.addictionpolicy.org/opioid-overdose.*

Good instructions for how to use Narcan and similar products (and conduct rescue breathing) can be found on the website of the Partnership for Drug-Free Kids at *www.drugfree.org/article/overdose-response-treatment.*

Detailed training is also available at *www.getnaloxonenow.org.*

CRAFT TECHNIQUES

Some useful books that explain CRAFT techniques in detail are:

- *Beyond Addiction: How Science and Kindness Help People Change* by Jeffrey Foote et al. (Scribner, 2014).
- *Get Your Loved One Sober: Alternatives to Nagging, Pleading and Threatening* by Robert Meyers and Brenda Wolfe (Hazelden Publishing, 2013).
- *The Parent's 20 Minute Guide, Second Edition,* and *The Partner's 20 Minute Guide, Second Edition,* both by The Center for Motivation and Change (Lulu.com, 2016).

Parents who would like personalized coaching from another parent who is trained in CRAFT techniques can call the helpline of the Partnership for Drug-Free Kids. The number in the United States is (855) 378-4373.

INTERVENTIONS

You can find trained and certified interventionists in the United States on the website of the Association of Intervention Specialists at *www.associationofintervationspecialists.org/member*. A (small) list of Canadian members can be found at *www.associationofintervationspecialists.org/canada*, and a (small) list of U.K. members can be found at *www.associationofintervationspecialists.org/britain*.

The pioneering book written by the developer of the intervention idea, Vernon E. Johnson, is *Intervention: A Step-by-Step Guide for Families and Friends of Chemically Dependent Persons* (Hazelden Publishing, 1986).

A more recent and practical book on interventions is *Love First: A Family's Guide to Intervention* by Jeff and Debra Jay (Hazelden Publishing, 2008).

EMPLOYMENT LAW AND ADDICTION

In the United States

Detailed information on the Americans with Disabilities Act and addiction is available from the U.S. Commission on Civil Rights at *www.usccr.gov/pubs/ada/ch4.htm*.

A guide for employees to negotiating reasonable accommodations under the Americans with Disabilities Act is available from the U.S. Department of Labor at *www.askjan.org/Eeguide/index.htm*.

A guide to the Family and Medical Leave Act for employees and families, called *Need Time?*, is available from the U.S. Department of Labor at *www.dol.gov/whd/fmla/employeeguide.pdf*.

A guide to state family and medical leave laws and how they differ from the federal law can be found at *www.ncsl.org/research/labor-and-employment/state-family-and-medical-leave-laws.aspx*.

Outside the United States

Canada

The Canadian Human Rights Commission has published a booklet called *Impaired at Work* that discusses federal employment law and addiction. The booklet is intended for use by employers, but the information will be helpful to employees as well. It's available at *www.chrc-ccdp.gc.ca/sites/default/files/impaired_at_work.pdf*.

Most provinces also have their own laws and policies; a brief summary can be found at *http://employment.findlaw.ca/article/can-an-employer-fire-you-for-drug-or-alcohol-addiction*.

United Kingdom

The government has published a booklet outlining the law regarding drug use and employment, called *Drug Misuse at Work*. The booklet is intended for use by employers, but the information will be helpful to employees as well. It's available at *www.hse.gov.uk/pubns/indg91.pdf*.

Ireland

A summary of the relevant law is provided in a government publication called *Guide to Alcohol and Drug Misuse in the Workplace*, available at *www.drugsandalcohol. ie/20699/1/A-Guide-to-Alcohol-and-Drug-Misuse-in-the-Workplace-2010.pdf.*

A summary in question-and-answer format is available in another government publication called *Intoxicants at Work*, available at *www.hsa.ie/eng/Publications_and_Forms/Publications/Occupational_Health/Intoxicants_at_Work_Information_Sheet_.pdf.*

Another publication that may be useful is *Intoxicants in the Workplace*, written by a private law firm and available at *www.matheson.com/news-and-insights/article/intoxicants-in-the-workplace.*

Australia

The Australian Human Rights Commission has published a booklet for employers on the law regarding employees with a mental illness, called *Workers with Mental Illness: A Practical Guide for Managers*, which is available at *www.humanrights. gov.au/sites/default/files/document/publication/workers_mental_illness_guide_0.pdf.*

The Federal Court has held that opioid addiction is a disability for purposes of the Disability Discrimination Act of 1992 (*Marsden v. HREOC* [2002] FCA 1619.) A similar decision has been reached under the law of New South Wales. See *Addiction: Is It a Disability?*, published by a private law firm and available at *www.maddocks.com. au/addiction-disability.*

New Zealand

Employment New Zealand has published a guide called *Drugs, Alcohol and Work* that outlines employment law issues concerning addiction. It's available at *www.employment.govt.nz/workplace-policies/tests-and-checks/drugs-alcohol-and-work.*

DRUG COURTS

In the United States

The National Drug Court Resource Center lets you search for drug courts in your area and provides detailed contact information at *www.ndcrc.org/map*. The site also lets you search for specialized court programs (such as for juveniles, veterans, co-occurring disorders, etc.).

Outside the United States

Drug courts are newer and less common outside the United States, but their numbers are growing. They generally operate in the same way as in the United States, with minor variations.

Canada

Drug courts operate in Alberta, British Columbia, Manitoba, Nova Scotia, Ontario, and Saskatchewan. You can find links and more information at *www.cadtc. org/dtcs-canada*.

United Kingdom

Drug court programs are fairly common in England and parts of Wales and have been introduced more recently in Northern Ireland. Information from the College of Policing is available at *http://whatworks.college.police.uk/toolkit/Pages/Intervention. aspx?InterventionID=34*.

Ireland

A drug court program exists in Dublin. See *www.courts.ie/Courts.ie/library3. nsf/(WebFiles)/DA10E72CEB411A0E80257297005BD8C9/%24FILE/Drug%20Treatment%20Court%20-%20public%20info.pdf*.

Australia

Drug courts operate in:

- Queensland; see *www.courts.qld.gov.au/courts/drug-court*.
- New South Wales; see *www.drugcourt.justice.nsw.gov.au*.
- Victoria; see *www.magistratescourt.vic.gov.au/jurisdictions/specialist-jurisdictions/drug-court*.
- Adelaide; see *www.courts.sa.gov.au/OurCourts/MagistratesCourt/Intervention Programs/Pages/Drug-Court.aspx*.
- Perth; see *www.courts.dotag.wa.gov.au/d/drug_court.aspx*.

New Zealand

In New Zealand, drug courts are called "Therapeutic Courts." There are two in Auckland and one in Wellington. More information from the Ministry of Justice is available at *www.justice.govt.nz/courts/criminal/therapeutic-courts*.

CIVIL COMMITMENT FOR ADDICTION

In the United States

State-specific information on civil commitment requirements is available from:

- The National Alliance for Model State Drug Laws, at *www.namsdl.org/ IssuesandEvents/NEW%20Involuntary%20Commitment%20for%20Individuals%20with%20a%20Substance%20Use%20Disorder%20or%20Alcoholism%20 August%202016%2009092016.pdf*.
- LawAtlas, at *www.lawatlas.org/datasets/long-term-involuntary-commitment-laws*.

State laws change (and are often complicated) and these resources might not be complete or up-to-date; it's best to consult a lawyer or court official for the most current information.

For a very detailed article about civil commitment in the United States, see Megan Testa and Sara G. West, "Civil Commitment in the United States," at *www. ncbi.nlm.nih.gov/pmc/articles/PMC3392176*.

Outside the United States

Canada

In Canada, civil commitment is called "civil committal." Every province has a law allowing it. Typically, the standard is that the person has a mental disorder and presents a danger to self or others. Patients in most cases can be committed to a hospital for a few days, and much longer if two doctors feel it is necessary. Patients can then apply to a court and argue for release. Most such laws are called "Mental Health Acts," and you can generally find the relevant law online by searching for the name of the province and "Mental Health Act."

United Kingdom

The Mental Health Act allows civil commitment of people who have a mental disorder and ought to be detained in a hospital for their own health or safety or the safety of others. Except in emergencies, two doctors who are specialists or know the patient must agree. The initial detention can be 28 days but can be extended for much longer. More information from the NHS is available at *www.nhs.uk/NHSEngland/AboutNHSservices/mental-health-services-explained/Pages/TheMentalHealthAct. aspx.*

Ireland

Detailed information about civil commitment can be found at *www.citizensinformation.ie/en/health/health_services/mental_health/admission_to_a_psychiatric_hospital.html.*

Australia and New Zealand

A chart explaining civil commitment laws created by the Royal Australian and New Zealand College of Psychiatrists is available at *www.ranzcp.org/Files/ Resources/Mental-health-legislation-tables/1-Involuntary-commitment-and-treatment-comparing-m.aspx.*

Major changes in New Zealand law regarding civil commitment for addiction took effect in 2018. These changes are described at *www.health.govt.nz/our-work/ mental-health-and-addictions/preparing-commencement-substance-addiction-compulsory-assessment-and-treatment-act-2017.*

NEEDLE EXCHANGE PROGRAMS

In the United States

Directories of needle exchange programs are offered by:

- The North American Syringe Exchange Network, at *www.nasen.org/directory*.
- DetoxLocal (a private organization) at *www.detoxlocal.com/needle-exchanges*.

Outside the United States

Canada

Canada does not have a nationwide directory, but you can contact your local health authority for information.

A directory of Ontario programs can be found at *www.ohrdp.ca/find/find-a-needle-syringe-program*.

United Kingdom

Many needle exchange programs are run by pharmacies, so you can ask a local pharmacy or contact the NHS.

In Scotland, a directory of needle exchange programs can be found at *www.needleexchange.scot*.

Ireland

You can find needle exchange programs at *www.services.drugs.ie* by selecting "Needle exchange" under "Choose type of service" and then selecting a location.

The Irish Needle Exchange Forum offers additional information at *www.idpc.net/profile/irish-needle-exchange-forum*.

Australia

Needle exchange programs are run by pharmacies and specialized organizations. A government question-and-answer publication that explains them can be found at *www.health.gov.au/internet/main/publishing.nsf/Content/73934F5307F88EC7CA257BF0001E009F/$File/ques.pdf*.

In South Australia, you can search for a needle exchange program at *www.sahealth.sa.gov.au/wps/wcm/connect/public+content/sa+health+internet/health+services/drug+and+alcohol+services/clean+needle+program*.

New Zealand

You can find a needle exchange program at *www.nznep.org.nz/outlets*.

SAFE INJECTION SITES

Safe injection sites, where intravenous drug users can inject in a medically controlled environment, operate in Canada, Australia, and seven European countries (Denmark, Germany, Luxembourg, the Netherlands, Norway, Spain, and Switzerland). In the United States, they have been proposed in New York City, Philadelphia, and San Francisco.

Canada

In Vancouver, the InSite program can be found at *www.communityinsite.ca.*

In Montréal, a site operated by a group called Spectre de Rue can be found at *www.spectrederue.org/sis.*

Australia

In Sydney, the Uniting site can be contacted at *http://uniting.org/who-we-help/ for-adults/sydney-medically-supervised-injecting-centre.*

ADDICTION AND THE BRAIN

A detailed definition and explanation of addiction can be found on the website of the American Society of Addiction Medicine at *www.asam.org/resources/ definition-of-addiction.*

Information and research on a large variety of drugs and how they work can be found on the website of the National Institute on Drug Abuse at *www.drugabuse. gov/drugs-abuse.*

Extensive research on alcoholism can be found on the website of the National Institute on Alcohol Abuse and Alcoholism at *www.niaaa.nih.gov.*

Current research on co-occurring disorders and addiction can be found on the website of the National Institute on Drug Abuse at *www.drugabuse.gov/related-topics/ comorbidity.*

Addiction's effect on the brain at the biochemical level is discussed in more detail in James D. Stoehr, *The Neurobiology of Addiction* (Chelsea House Publishers, 2006).

Notes

CHAPTER 3

For a more technical but still readable explanation of the addiction process, see James D. Stoehr, *The Neurobiology of Addiction* (Chelsea House, 2006).

"Studies with laboratory rats have shown . . ." See, for example, G. Di Chiara and A. Imperato, "Drugs abused by humans preferentially increase synaptic dopamine concentrations in the mesolimbic system of freely moving rats," *Proceedings of the National Academies of Sciences of the United States of America*, 1988, 85(14), 5274–5278.

CHAPTER 4

The stress–vulnerability model was elaborated in the 1970s by J. Zubin and B. Spring. See "Vulnerability—a new view of schizophrenia," *Journal of Abnormal Psychology*, 1977, 86(2), 103–124.

The water tank metaphor comes from Mental Health Professional Online Development, a resource funded by the Australian government.

"A number of studies have confirmed that high levels of unrelieved stress tend to produce chemical changes in the brain that make mental illness more likely." See, for example, C. Goh and M. Agius, "The stress–vulnerability model: How does stress impact on mental illness at the level of the brain and what are the consequences?" *Psychiatria Danubia*, 2010, 22(2), 198–202; and S. Chetty et al., "Stress and glucocorticoids promote oligodendrogenesis in the adult hippocampus," *Molecular Psychiatry*, 2014, 19, 1275–1283.

"These studies show that if one twin becomes an addict, there's a much higher likelihood that an identical twin will become an addict than that a fraternal twin will." C. A. Prescott and K. S. Kendler, "Genetic and environmental contributions to alcohol abuse and dependence in a population-based sample of male twins," *American Journal of Psychiatry*, 1999, 156(1), 34–40. See also M. A. Enoch and D. Goldman, "The genetics of alcoholism and alcohol abuse," *Current Psychiatry Reports*, 2001, 3(2), 144–151; and D. W. Goodwin, "Alcoholism and genetics: The sins of our fathers," *Archives of General Psychiatry*, 1985, 42, 171–174.

"Other studies of adopted children have shown that children are more likely to become addicts if one of their birth parents was an addict than if one of their adoptive parents was an addict." See Deborah Hasin et al., "Genetics of substance use disorders," in William R. Miller and Kathleen M. Carroll, *Rethinking Substance Abuse* (Guilford Press, 2006), 69.

"For instance, scientists have been able to isolate certain genetic combinations that are more or less common in alcoholics and cocaine addicts. They have also been able to show that mice bred with certain genetic combinations respond very differently to drug stimuli." See, for example, Learn.Genetics, "Genes and addiction," at *http://learn.genetics. utah.edu/content/addiction/genes.*

"Many Asian people have a genetic enzyme variant that causes unpleasant reactions when they drink alcohol." See R. F. Suddendorf, "Research on alcohol metabolism among Asians and its implications for understanding causes of alcoholism," *Public Health Reports,* 1989, 104(6), 615–620.

"Naltrexone, which is sometimes given to recovering alcoholics to reduce cravings, works more or less well depending on the person's genetic makeup." See J. E. McGeary et al., "Genetic moderators of naltrexone's effects on alcohol cue reactivity," *Alcoholism: Clinical and Experimental Research,* 2006, 30(8), 1288–1296.

"In two otherwise similar geographic areas, if one has a higher density of bars and liquor stores, it will also have a higher density of problem drinkers." See, for example, Carla Campbell et al., "The effectiveness of limiting alcohol outlet density as a means of reducing excessive alcohol consumption and alcohol-related harms," *American Journal of Preventive Medicine,* 2009, 37(6), 556–569.

"Monkeys who are exposed to a stressful environment are much more likely to become addicted to cocaine." See Regina Walker, "So, is addiction genetic? Or not?" *The Fix,* September 1, 2015, *www.thefix.com/Genetics-addiction-connection-regina-walker0901.*

For general information on the Adverse Childhood Experiences Study, see *www. cdc.gov/violenceprevention/acestudy.*

"One follow-up survey found that every single type of ACE correlates with a higher risk of alcoholism in later life." See Shanta R. Dube et al., "Adverse childhood experiences and personal alcohol abuse as an adult," *Addictive Behaviors,* 2002, 27(5), 713–725.

"People who reported five or more ACEs were 7 to 10 times more likely to develop an addiction." See Shanta R. Dube et al., "Childhood abuse, neglect, and household dysfunction and the risk of illicit drug use: The Adverse Childhood Experiences Study," *Pediatrics,* 2003, 111(3), 564–572.

"For instance, a study in Sweden . . ." See Maia Szalavitz, "Genetics: No more addictive personality," *Nature,* 2015, 522, S48–S49.

"One study found that people who had a parent who was an addict were eight times more likely to become addicts themselves." See K. R. Merikangas et al., "Familial transmission of substance use disorders," *Archives of General Psychiatry,* 1998, 55(11), 973–979.

CHAPTER 5

The books cited are Marc Lewis, *The Biology of Desire: Why Addiction Is Not a Disease* (Public Affairs, 2016) and Jeffrey Foote et al., *Beyond Addiction: How Science and Kindness Help People Change* (Scribner, 2014).

Other books arguing that addiction is not a disease because substance abuse is purely voluntary include Stanton Peele, *The Meaning of Addiction: An Unconventional View* (Jossey-Bass, 1985) and Theodore Dalrymple, *Romancing Opiates: Pharmacological Lies and the Addiction Bureaucracy* (Encounter Books, 2008).

Although there are reasonable arguments that addiction is not a disease, many arguments made in this vein appear to be based on a misunderstanding of the contemporary view of the nature of addiction. For instance, both Peele and Dalrymple cite studies showing that many soldiers who frequently used heroin in Vietnam were able to stop using it when they returned to the United States. But this argument assumes that everyone who uses heroin frequently is an addict. In fact, it's likely that many soldiers used heroin to escape the horrors of war but did not become addicted—just as many people use prescription painkillers following surgery but do not become addicted.

Another argument is that addiction must be voluntary because the initial decision to use a substance was voluntary. This might make sense if everyone who ever drank alcohol or used drugs automatically became an addict. However, many people deliberately choose to use alcohol or drugs but only unintentionally become addicted.

Dalrymple notes that many addicts were able to give up opium when the Chinese government threatened them with the death penalty for using it. But this argument assumes that if addiction is a disease, it completely takes away a person's free will—whereas in fact addiction merely *impairs* a person's free will, and many addicts are able to give up using, at least temporarily, if the consequences are severe enough. To use an analogy, a person who has a terrible flu might be able to drag herself out of bed and go to work if the alternative is getting fired, but this doesn't prove that there is no such thing as the flu.

CHAPTER 6

"Research using EEG monitoring has shown that nicotine can also act as a depressant." See Heather Ashton et al., "Stimulant and depressant effects of cigarette smoking on brain activity in man," *British Journal of Pharmacology*, 1973, 48(4), 715–717.

"Opioid prescriptions have skyrocketed in the United States, and opioid addiction has as well (with overdose deaths more than tripling between 2000 and 2016)." See the Centers for Disease Control and Prevention's Wide-Ranging Online Data for Epidemiologic Research, available at *http://healthdata.gov/dataset/wide-ranging-online-data-epidemiologic-research-wonder*. See also testimony of Dr. Nora D. Volkow before the Senate Caucus on International Narcotics Control, May 14, 2014, at *www.drugcaucus.senate.gov/sites/default/files/Volkow%20Testimony.pdf*.

CHAPTER 7

For a general review of similarities between substance and process addictions, see Jon E. Grant, "Introduction to behavioral addictions," *American Journal of Drug and Alcohol Abuse*, 2010, 36(5), 233–241.

"Substance abusers are 4 to 10 times more likely than the general population to have a gambling problem. This is especially true for people who are addicted to heroin and cocaine." See D. Ledgerwood and K. Downey, "Relationship between problem gambling and substance use in a methadone maintenance population," *Addictive Behaviors*, 2002, 27, 483–491; and B. Spunt et al., "Pathological gambling and substance misuse: A review of the literature," *Substance Use and Misuse*, 1998, 33(13), 2535–2560.

"Most often the substance abuse happens first, but sometimes it's the other way around, and sometimes both problems start at the same time." See O. Kausch, "Patterns of substance abuse among treatment-seeking pathological gamblers," *Journal of Substance Abuse Treatment*, 2003, 25, 263–270.

"In psychological tests, people with OCD tend to score low on impulsivity and high on the desire to avoid harm to themselves, whereas people who have process addictions are often just the opposite." See Jon E. Grant, "Introduction to behavioral addictions," *American Journal of Drug and Alcohol Abuse*, 2010, 36(5), 233–241.

CHAPTER 10

The books cited are Elisabeth Kübler-Ross, *On Death and Dying: What the Dying Have to Teach Doctors, Nurses, Clergy and Their Own Families*, 40th anniv. ed. (Routledge, 2008); Robin Norwood, *Women Who Love Too Much: When You Keep Wishing and Hoping He'll Change* (Pocket Books, 2008); and Melody Beattie, *Codependent No More: How To Stop Controlling Others and Start Caring For Yourself*, 2nd rev. ed. (Hazelden, 1992).

"An interesting study by a Stanford University professor . . ." Research by Rudolf Moos cited in David Sheff, *Clean: Overcoming Addiction and Ending America's Greatest Tragedy* (Houghton Mifflin Harcourt, 2013), 109.

CHAPTER 12

"Statistics show that addiction treatments can be quite successful even if the addict hasn't freely chosen to participate." See, for example, M. Douglas Anglin et al., "The effectiveness of coerced treatment for drug-abusing offenders," paper presented at the Office of National Drug Control Policy's Conference of Scholars and Policy Makers, March 23–25, 1998, available at *www.ncjrs.gov/ondcppubs/treat/consensus/anglin.pdf*.

"There have been a handful of scientific studies regarding the effectiveness of CRAFT." For a review, see Robert J. Meyers, Hendrik G. Roozen, and Jane Ellen Smith, "The Community Reinforcement Approach: An update of the evidence," *Alcohol Research and Health*, 2011, 33(4), 380–388, available at *www.ncbi.nlm.nih.gov/pmc/articles/PMC3860533*.

CHAPTER 13

"A 2006 survey conducted by Al-Anon of its members in the United States and Canada showed that 85 percent were women." See Al-Anon Family Groups, *Member Survey Results, Al-Anon Family Groups, Fall 2006*.

CHAPTER 14

"Research shows that the most common age for the onset of alcoholism is 18 to 19. It's certainly possible to develop the problem earlier or later, although statistically the likelihood decreases significantly after age 25." See Yann Le Strat et al., "A new definition of early age at onset of alcohol dependence," *Drug and Alcohol Dependence*, 2010, 108(0), 43–48.

"As for opioids, one study found that the average age of first use is between 25 and 26." See Leen Naji et al., "The association between age of onset of opioid use and comorbidity among opioid dependent patients receiving methadone maintenance therapy," *Addiction Science and Clinical Practice*, 2017, 12, 9.

CHAPTER 16

"U.S. government figures show that misuse of alcohol and prescription drugs by the elderly is one of the fastest-growing health problems in the country and affects as many as 17 percent of people over age 60." See U.S. Department of Health and Human Services Substance Abuse and Mental Health Services Administration, "Chapter 1: Substance abuse among older adults: An invisible epidemic," in *Substance Abuse among Older Adults*, October 2012, available at *www.ncbi.nlm.nih.gov/books/NBK64422*.

"One study found that among women over 60 in the United States, binge drinking increased at an average rate of 3.7 percent per year between 1997 and 2014." See Rosalind A. Breslow et al., "Trends in alcohol consumption among older Americans: National Health Interview Surveys, 1997 to 2014," *Alcoholism: Clinical and Experimental Research*, 2017, 41(5), 976–986.

The book cited is Janet Woititz, *Adult Children of Alcoholics*, 2nd exp. ed. (HCI, 1990).

CHAPTER 17

The case involving the assistant fire chief in Lima, Ohio is *DePalma v. City of Lima*, 155 Ohio App. 2d 81, 799 N.E.2d 207 (2003).

The case involving the freight company driver is *Ostrowski v. Con-way Freight, Inc.*, No. 12-3800, 2013 WL 5814131, 2013 U.S. App. LEXIS 22091 (3d Cir. Oct. 30, 2013).

CHAPTER 18

"Today there are more than 3,000 such programs across the United States, according to the National Association of Drug Court Professionals." See *www.nadcp.org/about*.

"Drug court programs have also been established in Australia, Belgium . . ." See *www.calgarydrugtreatmentcourt.org/international-results*.

"The U.S. Department of Justice has published figures showing that people who go through drug-court programs often have dramatically lower recidivism rates than other defendants." See *www.nij.gov/topics/courts/drug-courts/pages/work.aspx*.

For the statistics on the results of the Gloucester police program, see Shafaq Hasan, "One year later: Gloucester's opioid program inspires policy reform," *Nonprofit Quarterly*, June 3, 2016.

"Within a little over a year, some 160 other police departments across the country had created similar programs." See Ray Lamont, "Lawyer looks to ease cops' 'angel' burden with program changes," *Salem News*, October 10, 2016.

For William Fitzpatrick's comments, see Douglass Dowty, "Syracuse DA blasts police-run heroin amnesty programs on national television," *Syracuse Times*, June 6, 2016.

"In fact, a 2016 law review article . . ." See Grace Panetta, "The opiate crisis: Shifting discretion from prosecutors to police," *Columbia Undergraduate Law Review*, August 31, 2016.

The New Jersey Supreme Court case is *State v. Patton*, 133 N.J. 389, 627 A.2d 1112 (1993). See also *State v. Novak*, No. A-5841-08T45841-08T4 (NJ App. Div. Feb. 22, 2010) (applying *Patton* to facts more similar to a police amnesty case). These cases do not say that a person who voluntarily turns drugs over to police can never be prosecuted for possession; they say that if a person voluntarily turns drugs over to police, this fact cannot be used as evidence against him or her. Charges could still be brought if police have enough other evidence. Thus, while the cases would protect someone in the typical police-amnesty situation, where an addict goes to a police station and asks for help, they would not protect a drug user who is caught by law enforcement and *then* gives the drugs to the arresting officers.

CHAPTER 19

"The U.S. Supreme Court ruled that it was unconstitutional for the government to make it a crime to be an addict." See *Robinson v. California*, 370 U.S. 660 (1962).

For statistics on the frequency of civil commitment proceedings by state, see Christopher et al., "Nature and utilization of civil commitment for substance abuse in the United States," *Journal of the American Academy of Psychiatry and the Law*, 2015, 43(3), 313–320, available at *http://jaapl.org/content/43/3/313.full*.

"Only seven states specifically prohibit civil commitment for addiction." See Christine Vestal, "Support grows for civil commitment of opioid users," available at *www.pewtrusts.org/en/research-and-analysis/blogs/stateline/2017/06/15/support-grows-for-civil-commitment-of-opioid-users*.

For a discussion of the standards for civil commitment in various states, see Megan Testa and Sara G. West, "Civil commitment in the United States," *Psychiatry (Edgmont)*, 2010, 7(10), 30–40, available at *www.ncbi.nlm.nih.gov/pmc/articles/PMC3392176*.

The Supreme Court case adopting the "clear and convincing" standard is *Addington v. Texas*, 441 U.S. 418 (1979).

CHAPTER 20

For a review of U.S. state laws regarding ignition interlock devices, see *www.ncsl.org/research/transportation/state-ignition-interlock-laws.aspx*.

"Home urine tests . . . typically won't pick up very recent drug use, such as use within the last hour or two. With crack cocaine, heroin, and methamphetamines, it can take up to six hours before the drug can be detected in a person's urine, and with ecstasy and benzodiazepines, it can take up to seven hours." See U.S. Food and Drug Administration, "Drugs of abuse home use test," available at *www.fda.gov/MedicalDevices/ProductsandMedicalProcedures/InVitroDiagnostics/DrugsofAbuseTests/ucm125722.htm*.

For a review of studies regarding transcutaneous electrical nerve stimulation, see Vance et al., "Using TENS for pain control: The state of the evidence," *Pain Management*, 2014, 4(3), 197–209, available at *www.ncbi.nlm.nih.gov/pmc/articles/PMC4186747*. The article concludes, "The evidence for TENS efficacy is conflicting."

"Long-acting opioids may be preferable to short-acting ones because the 'high' produced by psychotropic drugs is usually related to the speed at which the concentration of the drug increases in the bloodstream." See Prater et al., "Successful pain management for the recovering addicted patient," *Primary Care Companion to the Journal of Clinical Psychiatry*, 2002, 4(4), 125–131, available at *www.ncbi.nlm.nih.gov/pmc/articles/PMC315480*.

CHAPTER 21

"President Bush said . . . he didn't believe he was 'clinically an alcoholic.'" See Lois Romano and George Lardner, Jr., "Bush's life-changing year," *Washington Post*, July 25, 1999.

CHAPTER 24

"The results are mixed . . . research has shown that the people who go to outpatient programs tend to be a very different population from those who go to residential programs." See Gregory B. Collins, "Emerging concepts of alcoholism treatment: Challenges and controversies," in Norman S. Miller, ed., *The Principles and Practice of Addictions in Psychiatry* (Saunders, 1997).

CHAPTER 25

The book cited is Anne M. Fletcher, *Inside Rehab: The Surprising Truth about Addiction Treatment—and How to Get Help That Works* (Viking Press, 2013).

The 2008 law is the Mental Health Parity and Addiction Equity Act, Pub. L. No. 110-343, 122 Stat. 3765, H.R. 1424.

The "Affordable Care Act" is the Patient Protection and Affordable Care Act, Pub. L. No. 111-148, 124 Stat. 119 (2010), as amended by the Health Care and Education Reconciliation Act, Pub. L. No. 111-152, 124 Stat. 1029 (2010).

CHAPTER 26

"Research suggests that MET is more effective with alcohol and marijuana than with heroin or cocaine." See the National Institute on Drug Abuse's *Principles of Drug Addiction Treatment: A Research-Based Guide* (3rd edition), available at *www.drugabuse. gov/publications/principles-drug-addiction-treatment-research-based-guide-third-edition/ evidence-based-approaches-to-drug-addiction-treatment/behavioral-2*.

CHAPTER 27

In 2010, a doctor named Olivier Ameisen published a book called *The End of My Addiction: How One Man Cured Himself of Alcoholism* (Piatkus Books), in which he claimed that he eliminated his alcoholic cravings by giving himself high doses of the muscle relaxant baclofen. However, more recent scientific studies have cast doubt on baclofen's effectiveness as an alcoholism treatment. See, for example, "Baclofen is largely ineffective for alcohol use disorders, finds study," *British Medical Journal*, 2018, 360.

CHAPTER 28

"A 2018 study sponsored by the National Institute on Drug Abuse . . ." See "Comparative effectiveness of extended-release naltrexone versus buprenorphine-naloxone for opioid relapse prevention (X:BOT): A multicentre, open-label, randomised controlled trial," *The Lancet*, January 27, 2018, 309–318.

CHAPTER 29

"Some doctors who advocate psychotherapy as a primary treatment have cited these latter statistics in an attempt to debunk AA." See, for example, Lance Dodes, *The Sober Truth: Debunking the Bad Science Behind 12-Step Programs and the Rehab Industry* (Beacon Press, 2014).

"A study led by a Harvard Medical School professor showed that attending AA meetings can significantly reduce symptoms of depression." See "Attendance at Alcoholics Anonymous meetings may reduce depression symptoms," available at *www.massgeneral.org/psychiatry/news/pressrelease.aspx?id=1200*. The professor commented, "Some critics of AA have claimed that the organization's emphasis on 'powerlessness' against alcohol use and the need to work on 'character defects' cultivates a pessimistic world view, but this suggests the opposite is true."

CHAPTER 31

"One study published in 2018 . . ." See "A longitudinal study of the comparative efficacy of Women for Sobriety, LifeRing, SMART Recovery, and 12-step groups for those with AUD," *Journal of Substance Abuse Treatment*, 2018, 88, 18–26.

CHAPTER 32

"According to U.S. government figures from 2014 . . ." See the U.S. Department of Health and Human Services Substance Abuse and Mental Health Services Administration 2014 National Survey on Drug Use and Health, available at *www.samhsa.gov/data/sites/default/files/NSDUH-FRR1-2014/NSDUH-FRR1-2014.pdf*.

"Although antisocial personality disorder is rare, alcoholics are 21 times more likely to have it than the average person—whereas they are no more likely to have an anxiety disorder than the average person." See J. E. Helzer and T. R. Pryzbeck, "The cooccurrence of alcoholism with other psychiatric disorders in the general population and its impact on treatment," *Journal of Studies on Alcohol*, 1988, 49(3), 219–224.

"A person with an anxiety disorder is twice as likely as the average person to develop an addiction of some sort." See studies cited at *www.drugabuse.gov/sites/default/files/rrcomorbidity.pdf*.

"One study has suggested that drug addicts are more likely than alcoholics to have an additional mental illness, although the figures are high for both groups." See D. A. Regier et al., "Comorbidity of mental disorders with alcohol and other drug abuse. Results from the Epidemiologic Catchment Area (ECA) Study," *Journal of the American Medical Association*, 1990, 264(19), 2511–2518.

"Among people with schizophrenia, the rate of smokers has been reported to be as high as 95 percent." See Nora D. Volkow, "Addiction and co-occurring mental disorders," *National Institute on Drug Abuse Notes*, February 1, 2007, available at *www.drugabuse.gov/news-events/nida-notes/2007/02/addiction-co-occurring-mental-disorders*.

CHAPTER 33

"One study showed that single women who become romantically involved with someone in the first three months of recovery are five times more likely to relapse than single women who don't." Judith A. West, "The Prince Charming syndrome," 1983 PhD dissertation cited in James W. West, *The Betty Ford Center Book of Answers* (Pocket Books, 1997).

CHAPTER 34

"Even seeing a picture of something associated with drug use—such as a syringe or a mound of white powder—can cause a sudden release of dopamine in the nucleus accumbens." See Linda Carroll, "Genetic studies promise a path to better treatment of addictions," *New York Times*, November 14, 2000.

"Images relating to cocaine use could trigger a dopamine reaction in the brain even though addicts were exposed to them for only 33 thousandths of a second." See A. R. Childress et al., "Subconscious signals can trigger drug craving," *Science Daily*, February 6, 2008.

"One of the most commonly cited statistics, . . ." See the National Institute on Drug Abuse's *Principles of drug addiction treatment: A research-based guide* (third edition), available at *www.drugabuse.gov/publications/principles-drug-addiction-treatment-research-based-guide-third-edition/evidence-based-approaches-to-drug-addiction-treatment/behavioral-2*, and *Drugs, brains, and behavior: The science of addiction*, available at *www.drugabuse.gov/publications/drugs-brains-behavior-science-addiction/treatment-recovery*.

CHAPTER 35

"A study conducted in 1998 found that as many as 90 percent of alcoholics were smokers." Research cited in David J. Drobes, "Concurrent alcohol and tobacco dependence," National Institute on Alcohol Abuse and Alcoholism, November 2002.

"A 2008 survey found that 57 percent of recovering alcoholics who participated in AA smoked." See Peter R. Martin et al., "Coffee and cigarette consumption are high among AA attendees," *Alcoholism: Clinical and Experimental Research*, October 2008.

"There's research suggesting that treating people for alcoholism and nicotine addiction at the same time is beneficial." See, for example, R. D. Hunt, K. M. Eberman, et al., "Nicotine dependent treatment during inpatient treatment for other addiction," *Alcoholism, Clinical and Experimental Research*, 1994, 18.

"In recent years a large number of scientific studies have demonstrated the effectiveness of this approach." See the studies cited in Christian S. Hendershot et al., "Relapse prevention for addictive behaviors," *Substance Abuse Treatment, Prevention, and Policy*, 2011, 6, 17, available at *https://substanceabusepolicy.biomedcentral.com/articles/10.1186/1747-597X-6-17*.

"At least one scientific study has shown that MBRP is effective in reducing relapse rates." See Sarah Bowen et al., "Mindfulness-based relapse prevention for substance use disorders: A pilot efficacy trial," *Substance Abuse*, 2009, 30(4), 295–305.

CHAPTER 36

"There are scientific studies that back up this view." See research cited in G. Alan Marlatt and Katie Witkiewitz, "Relapse prevention for alcohol and drug problems," in G. Alan Marlatt and Dennis M. Donovan, eds., *Relapse Prevention*, 2nd ed. (Guilford Press, 2005).

Index

About the Authors

Thomas F. Harrison is a professional writer and the former editor of a national periodical for attorneys. After a close friend developed a substance use problem, he devoted himself to helping families and friends learn how to cope with the challenges of addiction. He is based in Cambridge, Massachusetts.

Hilary S. Connery, MD, PhD, is Clinical Director of the Division of Alcohol and Drug Abuse at McLean Hospital in Belmont, Massachusetts, and Assistant Professor of Psychiatry at Harvard Medical School. An expert clinician and researcher, Dr. Connery has worked to educate family members and involve them in treatment since entering clinical practice in 2000.